TORCH

Tales Of Remarkable Courage And Hope

By Ovarian Cancer Survivors

Virginia R. Cvetko
Patient Education Center

Baylor Charles A. Sammons
Cancer Center at Dallas

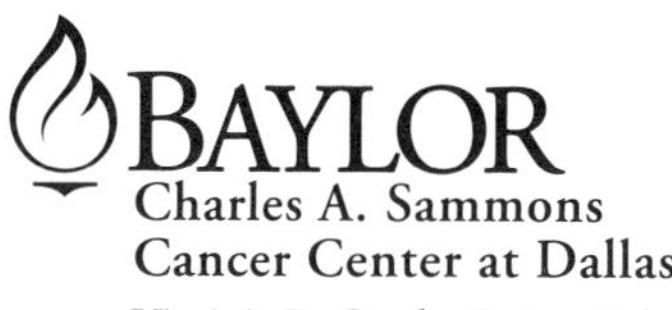

3535 Worth Street
Collins Suite 615
Dallas, Texas 75246
(214) 820-2608
BaylorHealth.com

Cover painting by Shannon Kincaid-Stringer

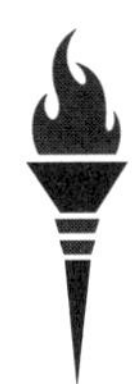

Dedication

TORCH, *Tales of Remarkable Courage and Hope*, is dedicated to those women who saw the need for a support group. These women founded this ovarian cancer support group and came faithfully during the early years. They sat and shared their stories with one another. By doing so, their courage was stiffened, and deep friendships were formed. They blazed a trail for those of us coming today. We feel deeply grateful to them for their example of courage and strength.

TORCH, Tales of Remarkable Courage and Hope, is dedicated to women who have been diagnosed with ovarian cancer. You are fighting the battle today. It is our hope that as you read our stories, your courage will be stiffened. This effort is dedicated to you.

TORCH, Tales of Remarkable Courage and Hope, is dedicated to those women who will be diagnosed. Over 20,000 will hear those words this year. We want you to know we are passing the torch of hope to you. Take hold, get a firm grip, hang on, don't let go, and never, never, never give up!

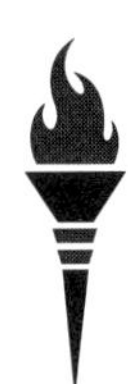

Table of Contents

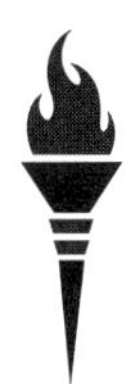

Acknowledgments

"WRITE A BOOK? Are you kidding?" That was the response of the ovarian cancer support group when the idea of *TORCH* was presented to them. "All I know is God said we're to write our stories and publish them as a book to encourage other ovarian cancer patients. We're to call it *TORCH, Tales of Remarkable Courage and Hope.*"

The first person we have to acknowledge for this effort is the Reverend Jann Aldredge-Clanton, an oncology chaplain at Baylor University Medical Center in Dallas, Texas. She was the first to hear the idea of a book. Her response was "This is a wonderful idea; we must do it." She could have pointed out all the barriers, obstacles, and negatives. She did just the opposite. She encouraged, supported, and promoted the idea. Not surprising, since she does that weekly at our group meetings. Jann has created a climate of love and acceptance for each of us as we seek to understand and be understood. We are beyond grateful to her!

"Thank you" seems so small in light of the big contribution Baylor University Medical Center makes to us individually and as a group. Driving up to the facility, we are met with huge banners proclaiming "Help Us Conquer Cancer." We get the feeling we have come to the right place. From the first people we encounter at the registration desk, we are met with smiles and friendliness that help relieve the stress of our visits. The lab techs are not only warm and welcoming, but they are also "good sticks," and we're grateful. Entering our beautiful meeting room in the basement, we feel as though we've come into someone's lovely living room. We have the Cvetko Patient Education Center to thank for that. They also provide lunch for us on the first

Monday of each month. Trays of sandwiches, fruits, and cheeses are laid out for us to enjoy. They also provide bottled water and lots of Kleenex. We've received spiral notebooks to use as journals and for note taking. They have also provided guest speakers who are experts in their field. Cvetko is an excellent resource for educational materials.

We are proud to have the medical director of the Virginia R. Cvetko Patient Education Center, C. Allen Stringer, MD, contributing his thoughts in our Foreword. Dr. Stringer came to Dallas in 1989 as the medical director for gynecology for Texas Oncology. Prior to this he held joint appointments at the University of Texas Medical School at Houston and M. D. Anderson Cancer Center. In 1993 he became chairman of the Department of Obstetrics and Gynecology at Baylor University Medical Center. In 1999 his interests in the psychological and psychosexual impact of a diagnosis of a gynecologic cancer were among the many reasons he began psychoanalytic training at the Dallas Psychoanalytic Institute, where he continues as an advanced candidate. In 2002 he became medical director of the Virginia R. Cvetko Patient Education Center. That year, he was also named a distinguished alumnus of the University of Texas Medical School at Houston. It is obvious from his education and experience that Dr. Stringer brings a wealth of knowledge to his patients, colleagues, and the Cvetko Center itself.

There are not words powerful enough to express our gratitude to all our doctors and nurses. They see us, truly, at our worst and sometimes at our best. Their efforts on our behalf surpass what one could expect. If the news is good, they are likely to be found dancing with us. If the news is not so good, we can see it in their eyes and hear it in their voices. They are healers and helpers in every sense of the word. It is overwhelming and humbling to be in their care. We each feel blessed beyond measure to have them.

One of the first "gifts" we were given for this book was Shannon Kincaid-Stringer. Shannon, a professional artist, heard about the project and offered herself and her talent. She created the cover of the book. When she brought her sketch to the group, we were breathless. We are still pinching ourselves at our good fortune. It is so like her that she continues to thank us.

Shannon did not stop with the artwork. She called with excitement about the possibility of writing a song. Her good friend, Steven Lawrence, came up with the most beautiful melody and lyrics. The day they came to the group to perform the song for us, we were grateful for Kleenex. The words, the music, and their love for us are deeply appreciated.

Our gratitude also goes to Shelley McClure, an exuberant member of the Cvetko Ovarian Cancer Support Group, for her generous contribution to the ongoing work of this Group. The McClure Fund helped make possible the publication of *TORCH*.

Thinking about those who have contributed to our project has taken us back to the beginnings of the group. Thirty years ago, in 1977, Virginia Cvetko and her good friend, Charlotte Barrett, started a cancer support group. That group continues to this day as a 6-week group for cancer patients. There have been over 100 groups to date. The 2-hour format allows for a guest speaker and a discussion time. Chaplains, other professional Cvetko staff members, and volunteers who are former members lead the groups. The Cvetko Patient Education Center opened in 1981. Ed Cvetko, Virginia's husband, and Bill Barrett, Charlotte's husband, are still involved. In January 1998, Dr. Stringer, Jann Aldredge-Clanton, and Billie Cope, an ovarian cancer patient, met. They discussed the need for an ovarian cancer support group. Ten years later, this book is a product of that group.

It goes without saying that our families and friends contribute daily to our health and well-being. Living with loving people makes such a difference, especially when we're battling cancer. They are loving, sometimes when we are not very lovable. We're tired, cranky, hurting, yet they're there with inspiring words such as "Bald is beautiful," "You have the loveliest-shaped head," and "The rain is no problem; if you want peach ice cream, I'll go get it." Often to their "What can I do to help?" we answer "Nothing." Having to accept that, to stand by while we struggle, must be terribly hard. Yet, they endure.

It is our prayerful desire that women who have been diagnosed with ovarian cancer will read this and feel encouraged and stirred to hope. We are passing on *TORCH*, our *Tales of Remarkable Courage and Hope*, to you. The passing of the torch is the critical part of a race. Please pass on the torch to someone else.

Becky Teter, Editor

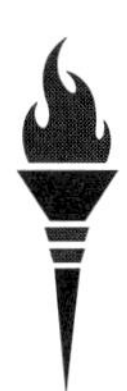

Foreword

IN THIS COLLECTION of stories by ovarian cancer survivors, you will read how women draw from their emotional and spiritual resources to complement the medical treatment they receive. This collection is aptly entitled *TORCH*, in that the women are passing the torch of hope to you. *TORCH* is also an acronym for *Tales of Remarkable Courage and Hope*. In my practice as a gynecologic oncologist, I am privileged to hear these remarkable tales and to see the stories unfold before me. The writers exemplify the strength of spirit and endurance that is so common in these patients.

As the medical director of the Virginia R. Cvetko Patient Education Center, it is my privilege to be in a position to educate and encourage patients who are diagnosed with malignant disease. The mission of the center is to give knowledge and hope to patients living with cancer. The members of the Cvetko Center staff include nurses, social workers, and chaplains who work as a multidisciplinary team to provide educational programs and support groups to cancer patients and their families. Virginia Cvetko, a breast cancer survivor, believed that doctors were not the sole owners of knowledge about a particular disease; rather, patients also possessed knowledge, and through group supportive activities this knowledge could be shared with others. Virginia was an intelligent woman and recognized the value of patients supporting one another. Her conviction led her to found the Self-Help Group, our first group and one that still meets today. This 6-week program consists of an hour of education on topics ranging from treatment modalities to coping strategies followed by an hour of group supportive therapy. The educational topics covered include diet, exercise, complementary therapies, sexuality, emotional responses, and spiritual resources. The group supportive therapy is led by a Cvetko Center professional staff member. It is vital that patients have information on those issues that will challenge them on their healing journey.

The approach used in the Cvetko Center is founded on the biopsychosocial model of treating the patient rather than the pure biomedical approach. According to the biopsychosocial model, the organic illness from which a patient is suffering has to be viewed in the context of the patient's emotional state and her or his social environment. The field of psychosocial oncology evolved from this philosophy and led to the adoption of a three-pronged approach to the care of the patient: education regarding the disease, development of coping strategies, and group supportive therapy. I have come to believe that the ability to maintain hope is essential for patients living with cancer. As caregivers, we must help our patients retain hope in the context of the reality of their situation. Hope that is unrealistic is just as destructive as hopelessness. Even when it is no longer realistic to hope for cure, there are many things for which the patient can remain hopeful. It is our job to help our patients identify and realize those goals.

Many ovarian cancer patients are uncomfortable in a group setting, especially early in the course of their illness. The more internal and external resources and support the patient has, the less likely she is to need group support. We have found, however, that a brief course of individual therapy allows many women who would otherwise not join a support group to transition into a group with beneficial results, including improved psychosocial adjustment and decreased anxiety.

I strongly encourage my patients to consider participation in a support group. The challenges resulting from a diagnosis of ovarian cancer can be overwhelming. Almost 10 years ago, Chaplain Jann Aldredge-Clanton, Billie Cope (a 12-year ovarian cancer survivor), and I sat down and discussed the need for an ovarian cancer support group. We started the group in conjunction with a research study that yielded preliminary results on the value of a support group to the quality of life of ovarian cancer patients. This pilot study served as a springboard for additional studies that have confirmed its value. The support group continues to grow in its outreach to women with ovarian cancer. This book is an effort by ovarian cancer survivors to reach out to women all across the country with the *TORCH* of hope.

I do believe we are on the cusp of major advances in the treatment of ovarian cancer. It is only a matter of time. There is great reason for hope.

C. Allen Stringer, MD
Medical Director, Virginia R. Cvetko Patient Education Center

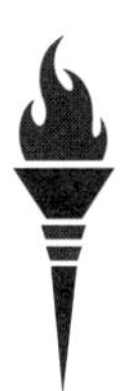

Introduction

IT IS 1:00 p.m. on Tuesday afternoon, January 9, 2007. My phone rings. It's Becky Teter, exclaiming, "I've just had a revelation while I was waiting in the take-out line at Whataburger! I see a torch, and women passing it on to other women! We're passing the torch through a book of our stories—you know, the women in the ovarian group writing our stories and publishing them in a book. And I see the title: *TORCH!* That's *T-O-R-C-H: Tales of Remarkable Courage and Hope.* We will pass the torch of hope to other ovarian cancer patients through telling our stories! What do you think?" My immediate response is, "Yes! What a great idea! I love the metaphor of the torch, and I know the power of stories. Go for it." The more I think about Becky's creative idea of a book of stories by women with ovarian cancer entitled *TORCH*, the more inspired it feels. If divine revelations can come in a burning bush and a manger, then why not in a Whataburger take-out line?

It is 11:30 on Monday morning, January 22, 2007. Women are gathering, as they do every week at this time, for a meeting of the ovarian cancer support group at Baylor University Medical Center. On this Monday morning, the women are celebrating the 17-year survival anniversary of Dody. The table in the center of the group displays 17 red roses and a chocolate cake with these words written in red icing: "Congratulations, Dody, on your 17th year of survival!" Dody sits resplendent—champagne blonde hair glowing, kind blue eyes twinkling, her whole being exuding hope and beauty. Women give her gifts of "17-something," like a necklace with 17 small light bulbs of many colors. We all pose for pictures with Dody.

Dody begins to tell her story of survival, from the day 17 years ago when she was diagnosed with stage III ovarian cancer to the present day. From her melodious southern voice flow the words "sweet" and "precious" over and over. She talks about how "sweet" and how "precious" these years have been and about how grateful she is for every day. She speaks about her gratitude to God also for giving her the opportunity to encourage other "girls" going through ovarian cancer. She acknowledges the difficult times she's been through. She tells of how her faith and her family and her friends have helped her through these rough times. But this is Dody's story, not mine, to tell. And you will read her story in her own words in this book.

I sit there listening to Dody's story and looking around the circle at the amazing group of women. As facilitator of the ovarian cancer support group, I have the holy privilege of hearing their stories of remarkable courage and hope. Each week these women inspire and challenge me. In this book you will read the stories of many of these women living with ovarian cancer. Like the stories told by the biblical writers, each story in this book reflects the unique personality of the writer. Some are direct and factual in telling their ovarian cancer stories, and others are expansive and expressive. Many of these stories have been told in the ovarian cancer support group. Telling their stories and hearing stories of others bring the women hope and encouragement.

Part of the existential search for meaning through the cancer experience is looking for patterns that give coherence to life. Telling their stories helps women with ovarian cancer in their search for meaning. Telling and hearing stories helps them integrate their current experience into their life stories in an effort to discover hope for the future. Through their stories they also explore things they may do with their ovarian cancer experience. The women offer these stories to you with the hope that they will help you through your ovarian cancer journey.

The narratives in this book hold sacred value. These stories reveal possibilities for human relationships and for relationship with the Divine.

> Story provides a pattern of meaning, coherence, and unity. The story is the primary vehicle for revealing who we are. Human experience is best portrayed as a narrative. A good story rings true, uniting us to what is sacred. It reminds us of our roots and challenges us to consider our destiny. It increases our capacity for reflection and empowers us to engage more fully in life. Wherever liberating action is happening, stories are being told. Our relationship to the divine is mediated through storytelling.[1]

Each week I witness the liberation that happens as the women in the ovarian cancer support group share their stories. I hear sighs of relief as one woman expresses feelings of fear that others are also feeling. Relief comes in having their feelings validated and normalized. Feelings buried to protect family members come pouring out, while heads nod in identification. A woman timidly expresses feelings she had been afraid to tell others because they might think she was "crazy." The others assure her with words and nods that they've had similar feelings. A woman tells a funny "bald head" story, and all the women laugh with relief. Women in the group find connection with one another as they speak and hear one another's stories. They free one another to accept their feelings as normal and to express their feelings. Releasing emotions that had weighed them down, the women find new freedom and energy for the healing journey.

Anne Lamott, in her book *Bird by Bird: Some Instructions on Writing and Life*, talks about writing books as presents to people.[2] These women have written the stories in this book as a gift to you, to bring you hope and encouragement through your ovarian cancer journey. These stories come to you as an invitation to find connections with your story and to see the holiness in your own story.

> We weave our lives with stories,
> blending
> > wide and narrow,
> > dull and bright,
> > dark and light,
> > joining
> the pieces with
> unending threads.
> Our stories link creation.
> Our stories bring revelation
> > of beauty unfolding
> > on a holy tapestry.[3]

Jann Aldredge-Clanton, PhD
Oncology Chaplain, Baylor University Medical Center

Notes

1. Conlon, J. *Earth Story, Sacred Story.* Mystic, CT: Twenty-Third Publications, 1994: 10, 16, 19.
2. Lamott, A. *Bird by Bird: Some Instructions on Writing and Life.* New York: Doubleday, 1994: 185–194.
3. Aldredge-Clanton, J. *Counseling People with Cancer.* Louisville, KY: Westminster John Knox Press, 1998: 40.

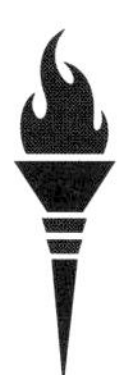

In God's Grace

I AM A STAGE IIIC ovarian cancer patient. The onset of this incident was so fast and serious that I still find it difficult to believe and accept. This year has been a tremendously eventful year of my life. When my eldest sister was diagnosed with stage III colon-rectal cancer back in July 2006, I was so sad in hearing the news. I took my two kids to visit her on December 24, 2006, in the hope of helping her out and cheering her up. However, I got sick and had a minor surgery in Vancouver while I was visiting her, and my ovarian cancer started popping up from December 27, 2006, onwards. My tummy began bloating up on and off until I looked like a 4-month pregnant lady.

My kids and I returned to Dallas on January 3, 2007. My other sister from Hong Kong was on a business trip and made a 2-day stopover to visit us from January 4 to January 6. She *insisted* that I must see a doctor on Monday. I know it's only been 14 days since this event began. Definitely, it was strange. I did see my family doctor on January 7, 2007, and was immediately referred to a gastroenterologist. The specialist immediately asked me to be admitted to the hospital for further testing. I stayed at the hospital for 3 days. The bad news came on the second day, especially when I started asking all the most difficult questions in my life. My ob-gyn told me on January 10 that she wanted me to have the surgery on January 15 by the gynecologic oncology surgeon. They needed to do a hysterectomy. Both of my ovaries were double the normal size of a 3- to 4-cm ovary, and there were images of tumors along the lining of the abdomen. In short, there were too many unknowns without opening me up to confirm where the rest of those obvious tumor cells were. Also, my blood test had such a high index for cancer cells, indicating that it was an advanced type of cancer. My index for the blood test of CA-125 was 1400. The normal range should be 0 to 35.

The question I asked my ob-gyn on the second day was "What is the prognosis for a stage IIIC ovarian cancer patient?" She wanted to defer the answer. But she was prepared enough to bring in a hospital nurse with her when she broke the news to me. She said that most ovarian cancer patients with a successful surgery may live for 4 or 5 more years. Hopefully, with the fact that I am younger than the statistical age group, perhaps I may have a better survival rate. I remember I was shaking my body on my chair, and I was sobbing so hard that I couldn't quite breathe or my sobbing was causing me to choke for a few moments. The nurse was so scared that she asked me if I would call my family before going further. But I moved on with my immense unbelievable mental pain inside me and asked if I could still be a normal mom to my kids after the hysterectomy surgery. By that time, I was so devastated that I deeply felt sorry for my two girls, Chantal and Gabrielle. How can they live without their mom!? How can I only have 4 or 5 more years left to love them and see them? *I want more!* I really want to see them growing up. They are only 5 and 6 years old....

Breaking the news to my family and friends was the way to release my intense emotional sorrow at that time. At the same time, I was trying to digest what God plans for me in all of this. A good friend and care provider for my younger girl encouraged me with this statement: "This is just a pretty make-up in disguise." I was encouraged because it is exactly what I wanted to understand, that everything works together for the glory of God. I did get something good out of such a bad circumstance. It is yet for me to discover and be reviewed by God in His time.

Now, I am searching to live beyond just *wanting* to be here for my girls— to do what is pleasing to God and to glorify Him. Not to mention, to be a better wife and to be a help to others in a special way, whether as an ovarian cancer patient, a mom, a wife, a friend, a neighbor, or whatever role I would be at that point.

Here comes the fun part. I told a few ladies at my ovarian cancer support group that this event is better than my wedding because three of my six siblings flew in one by one to give me the support that I have never experienced in my life. They arrived one after the other since I got out from my surgery on

January 19. They planned it so well that each one arrived with a 1- or 0-day overlap. Plus, all my friends whom I ask for help really enthusiastically give me "meals on wheels" without any questions. Some of my neighbors kept my two girls for a few nights during my surgery while my husband Len was with me at the hospital. Some of them sent them to school or picked them up for me. Not to mention the cards, the love, the flowers, the fruits, the gifts, the encouraging e-mails; the pastor who called to pledge his help or clients who felt speechless in hearing my news and wanted to love me; teachers who gave special attention to my girls during these times; and brand-new acquaintances of cancer survivors that came to tell me all the secrets about how to take care of myself, etc., etc.

I have never felt so much love before. The continuous visits from friends whom I haven't seen and friends who just want to help or care are amazing. I feel so blessed! God is really with me during all this. God definitely brings my family and friends closer than ever before. Yes, I am in His grace.

To update my situation, I had a port (a tube incised into the upper part of my left chest) done on February 12, 2007. It is still sore and painful. This is done for my next six chemotherapy sessions starting tomorrow. Even though I have still not recovered fully from my hysterectomy, the doctors and I have agreed not to wait any longer because I have the most aggressive cancer in my body. There are three types of cancer cells. I have type 3, which is the worst. This bad news gives me the good news that they tend to respond to chemotherapy better than type 1 or 2. Please pray for me that the cancer cells will respond well to the chemo so that they will all die. On the other hand, I need to have a good white blood cell count before every chemotherapy session. Please remember to fight with me together in your prayers. And I will pray for you and send you hope.

Olivia Chang

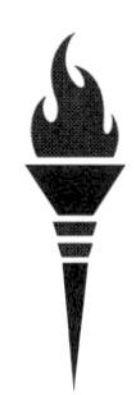

People Matter Most

A S IT TURNS OUT, my maternal grandmother was actually diagnosed with ovarian cancer at the age of 80. She died at 83; she'd been allergic to the chemotherapy. The family had never said "ovarian cancer." Instead, I was told colon or stomach cancer was the cause of her death. That might have been helpful to know when I was diagnosed in 2005. But let me go back 10 years.

I was working in the mortgage underwriting industry in 1993. There was a co-worker there named Dede. Through a series of circumstances, we were drawn to one another. The love of laughter, our work ethic, our ability to have deep and meaningful conversations sealed our commitment to each other. By 1995, we had begun a committed relationship that has endured to this day. We actually had 10 years of "life is good." Almost 10 years. In 2004, Dede's mother was diagnosed with melanoma. That fall, she had two surgeries. In early March 2005, Dede went out to stay with her mother. Her stay lasted for 45 days. During that time, she took care of her mother as she fought cancer. When she came home, we discussed our annual trip to the beach. I felt like I needed to stay but encouraged her to go. It was during that time that I decided to take my mother to a Texas Rangers' ballgame. We were both fans. Tickets to the game would make a great Mother's Day present.

I ordered the tickets over the Internet for Saturday, May 7, 2005. There was a mistake and the salesman called. He informed me he had sent the tickets, but they were one row behind what I ordered. He apologized, and I was fine with it. We were so excited to be going to the game. Texas was playing Cleveland. We were in Section 18, Row 7, seats 9 and 10. There were 48,000 people at the game. We were winning by several runs. We thought we might leave to go to the Mavericks playoff game. We were getting ready to go when Alfonso Soriano got up to bat. "Let's see if he hits another homer," I said. He'd already hit two. He swung and hit a line drive foul ball. It was going about 150 miles per hour when I realized it was heading straight for me. I couldn't move. It happened so fast.

The next thing I knew I was gasping for air, holding my stomach in serious pain. Little did I realize this would be the first miracle I would experience. The Rangers' first aid cart drove up. I was encouraged to go to an emergency room, but being concerned about my mother, I decided we'd just go home. The next day was Mother's Day, and we were at my sister's house. She's a nurse, and she insisted on seeing my stomach. I lifted my shirt. "You look like you're 9½ months pregnant," she said. We headed to the closest hospital in Fort Worth. The doctor ordered a CAT scan to see if the hit caused my spleen to burst or if there was kidney damage. Two scans were done. The doctor came in saying, "Well, the good news is your spleen is fine and the kidneys aren't damaged. But, you do have cancer." I couldn't believe it. Cancer? He had made an appointment with an oncologist. My sister said, "You can't say cancer when you've not done a biopsy." He said, "I know cancer when I see it."

The next morning we went to the oncologist's office. He confirmed what the emergency room doctor had said. I was admitted and a biopsy was done. Cancer. I got two other opinions. Dr. John Schorge at UT Southwestern Medical Center came highly recommended. He said, "It is stage IIIC ovarian cancer. You will need extensive surgery and chemotherapy." The surgery was done May 24, 2005. He found a large amount of cancer. A complete hysterectomy was done, removing 15 tumors; one alone weighed 10 pounds. My spleen was removed, as well as my appendix, a portion of my small intestine, and a large amount of fluid. I woke up 25 pounds lighter. On the third day following surgery, I had difficulty breathing. It became life threatening, and I was moved to the intensive care unit. I was there for 6 days.

A decision had to be made: to put me on a ventilator or not. I went on it and stayed 3 days. My second miracle was being able to breathe on my own. It happened on my mother's birthday. I then had eight rounds of chemotherapy, 3 weeks apart. A clear scan enabled me to become part of a phase III study. I received chemotherapy once a month with blood work weekly for 12 months. It was a maintenance plan to keep the cancer at bay.

Recently, I had a bout of what we thought was pancreatitis. I was hospitalized and treated with antibiotics and pain medication. Dede and I had been planning a trip to New York to the dog show. I wanted so badly to be able to go. Another miracle: we went. Not only went, but because of bad weather, we weren't able to fly back for 5 extra days. We had a ball. We arrived home, and I began to have some symptoms that required hospitalization. My doctor said, "Jenny, there is a tumor in the pancreas. It has its own blood supply. I recommend Avastin and Taxol. Avastin will kill its blood supply." Another miracle: a woman in my support group had been talking about Avastin. Her doctor was using it with her, off label. She was getting good results. I had decided to mention it. I didn't need to. My doctor suggested it. Now our prayer is that it works!

I feel it was *divine intervention* that directed that ball into my abdomen. That enabled the ovarian cancer to be found and treated. So much of what has happened has felt as though I have been led, guided, directed. I have to think God's been behind me all the way. And in front of me, too.

Ovarian cancer is called "the silent killer." You don't know you have it, usually, until it is advanced. There is no early detection test. We must be advocates. We must insist on more research. Part of my purpose now is to help educate women about this disease. I want to spread the word. There needs to be a solution. I am 44. I have much I want to do. I have people I love dearly: nieces and nephews and other family members I am not ready to say goodbye to. I am deeply grateful for this time to speak openly and boldly and often to those I love. I want my family to know how important they have been to me. I want them to know what's important: people matter. Relationships matter.

My support group is hoping that through telling our stories women who have received this diagnosis will be encouraged. We've been excited to watch this project come together. From the challenge to write to the beautiful painting for the book to the song that was written, this has been uplifting. This past Monday at our group meeting, the man who has written our song, "It Was You," came and sang it for us. As he sang the words, I was struck with the blessing of my partner, Dede. The song spoke of a "constant presence." That's Dede. She has not wavered. She has not weakened. I am very thankful to her and for her.

Jenny Sorrell

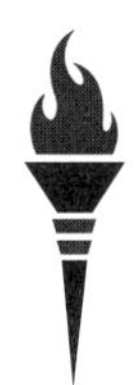

Yesterday, Today, and Forever

Yesterday He helped me; Today He did the same; How long will this continue? Forever, Praise His Name!

YEARS AGO, a dear friend gave me a wall plaque with the above words, and as I started on this journey, I would find these words to be true over and over again. I would never have chosen this journey, but I am thankful for all the things that I have learned along the way. God's Word has become more precious to me as I have learned to stand on His promises and apply them to my daily life. Each day is a gift as I walk this unknown pathway, but as promised, He is always by my side. Jesus is the one who brings peace into life's storms.

It was the summer of 2002, and I had just returned from my annual trip to the United Kingdom to visit my family. This had been my custom for the past 23 years, but my return this time would start a chain of unexpected events. I had not really felt well for a few months, but the possibility that I might have cancer had never entered my head. I had a persistent cough that I could not get rid of, and I was gaining weight, but I never thought it could be something serious. I joined Weight Watchers to lose what I later found out was a tumor. Obviously, I lost the targeted weight and then kept losing, not realizing that all the time the tumor was growing. I now jokingly say that I joined Weight Watchers to lose a tumor! It is important to keep a sense of humor even though at times there is not much to laugh about. At one stage it became too painful to laugh, so I would leave the room if something humorous was said.

Things moved quickly on my return to Dallas late one Saturday evening. Monday morning I was at my gynecologist's office. After examining me, with a very serious look on his face, he told me that I had a tumor and that things did not look good. The next day I had a series of tests at Baylor which confirmed my doctor's fears that I had a malignancy. Looking back at this time, I think I was in some kind of a bubble. I felt really sick and the thought that something was going to be done about it, even major surgery, was a relief. I seemed to take it all in stride at the time, but looking back I never really thoughtfully considered the seriousness of the diagnosis. I guess in some ways this was a blessing. My precious daughter and husband were right there with me. I think that the diagnosis was a lot harder on them because they realized what was ahead of me more than I did.

Two weeks after my surgery I started on chemotherapy and did not return to work for 6 months. To say that the months following were easy would not be truthful. I can say that I have never felt so loved and supported in all my life. I was overwhelmed by all the cards, flowers, visits, and food provided by my wonderful family, dear friends, church family, and colleagues at the office. What a comfort to know that so many people were praying for me and my family during our time of need! It was such an encouragement to know that others were standing in the gap for me when I was too weak to pray myself. On a follow-up visit with my oncologist after starting chemo, he asked me how I was feeling, to which I responded, "I am bald and blessed!" He said, "I guess you have lost your hair. Don't worry; it will grow back." And, of course, it did. I soon discovered that wearing a wig cut down on the time it took to get ready. It also saved money and time on trips to the beauty shop. Besides, I had other things to focus on than my hair!

My cancer has returned twice in less than 2 years since my original diagnosis, and consequently I have been more on chemo than off it. This is not a good prognosis for survival. However, I feel very blessed to be alive and attribute it to the excellent medical care I have received from my oncologists and the Great Physician's continued healing touch in my body.

There have been times when things did not look so good. One Thursday in December 2004, my oncologist referred me to a gastroenterologist because

I was unable to keep any food in my system. They were planning to have a tube inserted into my stomach the following week. I remember asking my oncologist if this would be permanent. He said that it could be removed, but somehow I had the impression that scenario was unlikely. I was feeling pretty rough during this time. On Sunday morning before that appointment, I had a strong desire to go to church, so with the help of my husband, I literally pushed myself to get there. I asked someone to let my pastor know that I was sick and wanted to be prayed for. At the end of the service I was anointed with oil and prayed for just like it says in James 5:14. By the time I saw the gastroenterologist on Wednesday I was feeling so much better and was able to eat again. The doctor opened the door to the room, looked in, and then left. A couple of minutes later he came back, asked me my name, and said, "Oh, I was looking for someone old and sick, and you look neither old nor sick!" After talking to me and examining me, he said, "Well, you are definitely not sick enough for a tube!" I explained to him that when I saw my oncologist I was in pretty bad shape, but that I was prayed for at church a few days earlier and had felt much better since. I knew this was an answer to prayer. He said, "I don't know about that, but you don't need me!"

I know through it all I have had the peace of God which surpasses earthly understanding. My faith has been tested and strengthened through this journey that I am still traveling. I know that no matter what happens, I am in the palm of His Hand. I have found there is no safer place to be.

It is just over 4½ years since my diagnosis. I have only recently visited, by accident, the ovarian cancer support group at Baylor. I regret that it took me so long to include this incredible group of remarkable women in my journey; they are traveling the same road. I am blessed to have found them, and I plan to make them a regular part of my life.

Muriel Ellis

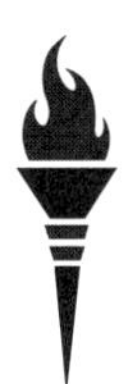

An Unexpected Journey

MY JOURNEY with ovarian cancer began nearly 4½ years ago in November 2002. Five months earlier, in May 2002, I decided to stop taking hormones because of the published cancer scares. About the same time, I noticed a gradual thickening around my middle. Attributing this to the fact that I was probably just going to get "fat" after no longer taking hormones, I put it out of my mind. In October, I started feeling a lot of discomfort in my upper abdomen, sort of a full feeling. Sometimes, when I sat down, I had trouble breathing, and my stomach was getting more and more chubby. However, I was not feeling any pain.

In late October 2002, I made an appointment with my family doctor who took one look at my bloated stomach and ordered a sonogram. Thankfully, because of his suspicions of ovarian cancer, he immediately ordered a CT scan that confirmed that I did have ovarian cancer. I know of so many heartbreaking stories where family practice doctors misdiagnose women with ovarian cancer. This is where my journey started in the right direction. I was then sent to a gynecologic oncologist, Dr. Bruce Fine, a most compassionate and thorough doctor. I will never forget that Friday afternoon in early November, a beautiful fall day in Texas. After Dr. Fine had a chance to look over my scan and read my CA-125 report, which indicated it was at 900, I asked him on a scale of one to ten how bad my cancer was. He answered a ten. I was diagnosed with stage IV ovarian cancer. I felt my knees weaken. Feeling suddenly nauseated, I hung my head over the exam room toilet with Jack, my husband, holding on to me. I felt totally numb. How could this be when I had been feeling so good? The reality was hard to fathom. My husband asked if we could come back Monday.

Dr. Fine, in no uncertain terms, told us to march across the street and check into Medical City. That was the longest walk of our 33 years of marriage.

Within 5 days, I had 7 hours of surgery. It was followed by several days in intensive care on a ventilator and a 3-week stay in the hospital, including a Thanksgiving "dinner." I was home in early December. A week after coming home, I started the usual regimen of six rounds of carboplatin and Taxol. My family and friends were simply amazing during this time. Friends cooked gourmet meals night after night and finished my Christmas shopping. One special friend even decorated my house from top to bottom, while Jack and our two grown daughters decorated the tree. It was magnificent! My parents had arrived before my surgery and stayed through Christmas. I really was overwhelmed by all of the love and kindness I felt that Christmas. It was the most meaningful Christmas I have ever had.

My treatment was successful, and after six rounds of chemotherapy, my CT scan showed no visible signs of cancer. Dr. Fine had encouraged me to participate in a clinical trial at M. D. Anderson. For me to be accepted into the trial, I had to have a "second-look" surgery to verify that I had no visible tumors. No tumors were found, just a few microscopic cells. So we were off to M. D. Anderson in Houston for the summer to continue my journey. The trial involved harvesting my stem cells, high-dose chemotherapy, followed by an autologous stem cell transplant. Dr. Fine felt the trial would give my cancer one more aggressive "blow"! The study was being run by Dr. Michelle Donato, a brilliant, compassionate young woman. I spent the summer in Houston and came home 2 days before our 34th wedding anniversary in early August 2003 to recuperate.

Following my transplant, I had three wonderful years of remission. Jack and I took many exciting trips and spent many special times with friends and family. Once I was feeling stronger, I decided to look into genetic testing. My mother had been diagnosed with stage I ovarian cancer in 1989. Not until I became sick did I possibly even think that I could have the *BRCA* gene that puts you at high risk for ovarian and breast cancer. I did, in fact, test positive for the *BRCA2* gene, as did my mother. Now my daughters had to make the decision of whether or not to be tested. They were both so brave and decided they wanted to know if they carried the gene. Paige, who was 32 at the time, tested negative. Brittney, who was 30, tested positive. It was such a difficult time for our family. But we all feel that knowledge is power, and we now have the knowledge we need to make the best decisions for our future. Brittney and I go for mammograms and sonograms every 6 months, and Brittney goes for her CA-125 and a vaginal sonogram every 6 months. Paige is also more diligent and aware because of her family history. We are so proud of both of them.

About the same time, I read an article in the paper about how two people met. The girl was Lora Williams. Lora was an ovarian cancer survivor. Her husband's mother had passed away from ovarian cancer, and that is what brought their two lives together. The article mentioned an ovarian cancer support group at Baylor that Lora was a part of. Up until then, I had never really thought I needed a "support group." I had all the support I needed with family and friends. But something drew me to the group, a sort of sisterhood. I am so thankful that my journey has brought them to me.

They have changed my life and enriched me in so many ways. Only "my sisters" can truly understand that once you are given a diagnosis of "cancer free," you are never truly free from cancer. It is with you every day. This wonderful group of ladies is the bravest I know. I listen to them tell their stories every Monday and am amazed by their strength. We laugh, we cry, and we share information. I have been traveling with them through our journey for 3 years, and they hold a special place in my life.

In July 2006, after three wonderful years of remission, my cancer returned. It was a 2-cm spot on my liver. Dr. Fine and Dr. Gogel performed surgery in August 2006, followed by six more treatments of carboplatin and Taxol. My treatments have been over now for 2 months. I had a clear PET scan in January, so once again I am in remission. I am feeling stronger every day. I am so excited about my new thick eyelashes and eyebrows and my fuzzy hair, even if it is gray. My husband has the sweetest way of kissing me on my head and rubbing the new sprouts of hair. He truly makes me feel that "bald is beautiful."

I feel very hopeful that I will have another long remission. As I look back on the last 4½ years of this unexpected journey, the road has been difficult, but it has also changed my life in so many positive ways. I have been carried along on my journey by my wonderful family, my very special friends, and the love of and strong belief in God.

Debby Sovern

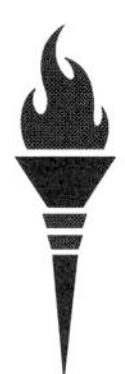

Bummer...

"**B**UMMER**"** was my comment to my husband upon learning my surgery revealed cancer. As I tried to awaken, surrounded by my husband, son, and two friends, I was not totally surprised. An intravaginal sonogram had revealed an abnormal, walled tumor on one ovary. Later I would learn my omentum, part of my bladder, and microscopic abdominal cells were also affected.

My recovery from surgery went well, and I felt great. As soon as I met with the gynecologic oncologist I said, "Let's get started with treatment." This would consist of six regimens of chemotherapy every 3 weeks. When I reacted to Taxol, we switched to Taxotere/cisplatin. I admit I feared nausea as much as anything. When the doctor prescribed some very expensive antinausea pills, I think I decided I would not be sick, and I wasn't. After the second treatment, I decided I could tolerate my two "dead days" every 3 weeks. Since I was working and quite healthy (except for cancer it seems), I worked during chemotherapy.

One of my friends was battling breast cancer, so she informed me about the wonderful medicine available to combat nausea, what to expect during chemo, and about wigs. Her advice was to buy a wig before I lost my hair. The doctor said I would lose it in about 2 weeks after chemo started. Nancy said my scalp would tingle or sort of hurt. Sure enough, the hair started coming out one Monday morning as I showered and prepared to go to work. That evening, I had my husband buy clippers and shave my head. It was a teary time!! I always said my head did not have a pretty shape and found it absolutely true. I kept telling myself it would grow back, and I did have that wig. The doctor said it would grow back but might be gray. When I asked if it had to stay gray, he said, "No." That made my day!

Helmets of hair—that's what wig designers make! There was so much hair in front! It reminded me of a bike helmet—or a really bad Elvis wig! My goal was to find a wig that was close in color and style to my existing hair. I finally found one and paid extra to have it styled. I did not need that entire bundle of hair in front. Most people, including my son, either did not know or forgot I was wearing a wig.

Perhaps I am just vain, or because I am a professional interior designer, I did not want to give cancer a "face." With my wig, clothing, and makeup, I satisfied that for myself. Thus, I felt more normal or better. Working during chemo kept me focused on something other than cancer. I realize I was lucky. My energy level was pretty good.

I started attending the ovarian cancer support group at Baylor while still recovering from surgery. I was afraid it would be depressing, but I could quit if I found that to be true. It has been an inspiration to me to see the courage, the hope, the prayers, and certainly the humor of these wonderful women. I felt a bit guilty because I thought I was stage I. I did question that since I spoke for the National Ovarian Cancer Coalition and their slides indicated I was at least a stage II. Fancy my surprise when I was denied some insurance because I was stage III and "not 5 years out"! I called my gynecologic oncologist's office to see what was going on. (I was seeing one of the other doctors in the group since my original doctor was out on leave.) Yep, stage III. Boy, I certainly felt better when I thought I was stage I! It was rather like being newly diagnosed.

Cancer is such a terrible disease. Far too often ovarian cancer is not diagnosed until it is stage III or IV. I hear the horror stories of the ladies in my group about months of complaining to a doctor regarding symptoms, which may be subtle and "normal"—bloating, gas, and fatigue.

My hope is that women will learn these subtle symptoms and will insist on further investigation by their doctor or another. It is up to all of us who have or will go through ovarian cancer to get the message out so those stats will become lower for late diagnosis.

The diagnosis *is* a bummer…but there is *hope*.

Jeannine Bazer Schwartz

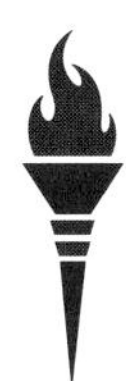

One in a Hundred

MY HUSBAND had retired and had just gotten used to working out of his office at home when I got the news that I needed some routine hernia repair. The surgery became not so routine when they decided the elongated knot in my groin was too hard to be a hernia and my CA-125 was elevated, which can indicate a tumor, cancer, or endometriosis. On Monday, September 8, 2003, the surgeon removed the knot and the nerve it was wrapped around, which would cause numbness in that area. That sounded pretty good to me since it had caused a lot of pain and some sleepless nights due to the nerve being involved. Because of the elevated CA-125 the surgeon did some laparoscopic work and found that there was a cancerous tumor on the backside of the uterus going down to the colon. It appeared to be very aggressive. My husband asked, "You have caught it early?" The surgeon, who had become a dear friend, reluctantly said, "No," and his tone did not give us much hope.

He referred me to a gynecologic oncologist. The appointment was 10 days away. I asked to be called if there were any cancellations. They informed me that I was very fortunate to get in the next week since the doctor's schedule was very full. I told them I appreciated what they were doing and then repeated my request. Sure enough that afternoon I received a call. The doctor would see me the next day, which was Friday.

In the space of about 3½ years, my husband and I lost seven family members and numerous dear friends. When I received the diagnosis, I had become resigned to the fact that it was probably now my time. But on Friday, I woke up with the realization that the Lord went to an awful lot of trouble for my cancer to be found even at an advanced stage. He had even arranged for this oncologist to have an opening to see me. This gave me new hope—a hope that God would heal me.

The oncologist was a gentle and thorough man who assured me he would do everything possible to treat this cancer. My husband showed him the pictures taken during the laparoscopic procedure. He asked the doctor to show him the cancer. The doctor said "the white stuff." That was not too comforting because most of the pictures were "the white stuff." More tests were scheduled for Sunday, since that was the first available date. He wanted to get my records from the previous lab work. The oncologist also expressed a sincere statement about how pleased he was that he had been able to see me so soon. My husband asked the doctor, "What is the outlook?" The doctor replied, "There are women who have been this sick and are out there walking around cured. You concentrate on that." My husband said that was not too encouraging at the time, but he now feels it was the best advice he could have had.

After the doctor completed his evaluation and informed me of all my options, I decided to go with his recommendation of three rounds of chemotherapy before surgery. We hoped the cancer would pull back and I would not have to have a bowel resection, which appeared to be inevitable if we did the surgery first.

My husband went with me to look at wigs. It was a certainty I would need one some time between the first and second treatment. Well, I looked at everything and could not decide on anything. My husband just calmly made the statement, "We are not leaving the store until you pick one." With his help, I did. I was so grateful I had it when all my hair came out. Just put that thing on and if the body was willing, I was ready to face the world.

In the waiting room I had mixed emotions about my first chemotherapy that I would be receiving shortly. The Lord brought two special passages to my attention. The first was Jeremiah 31:3–4. The Lord is speaking: "I have loved you with an everlasting love, I have drawn you with loving-kindness. I will build you up again." The second was Jeremiah 31:16: "Restrain your voice from weeping and your eyes from tears, for your work will be rewarded, declares the Lord." He is so faithful to bring us strength as we keep looking to Him. The first chemo was extremely painful for several days, but I took heart when the doctor explained that the chemotherapy might really be dealing the cancer a crippling blow. That helped make the sleepless nights more bearable.

There were times my legs, feet, and hands got so painful it was difficult to sleep, but lots of different pillows and odd positions would help sometimes.

My oncologist had encouraged me to take part in a trial support group that he was involved with. I signed papers to attend this ovarian cancer support group. I would fill out some evaluation papers from time to time. I was afraid I was not going to be able to handle it. I thought it might make me depressed. My doctor assured me that if, at any time, I felt it was hurting me, I should stop. If he thought it was having an adverse effect on me, he would pull me out. What a blessing in disguise this group was and still is. All those questions you were afraid to ask or thought your friends wouldn't understand could be shared. Experts were brought in so we might ask questions and learn. There are things you don't want to burden your friends and family with, but you realize other ovarian cancer patients are going through the same thing. What a blessing these women have been in my life. They are wonderful friends and exceptional ladies.

After three rounds of chemotherapy, I had my surgery. Now we would find out how well the cancer responded to the treatment. The wait was worth it. The chemo had been effective. The hysterectomy was done, the tumor removed, and a few other things deemed necessary. And, of course, the debulking (just think, a few months ago I had no idea what debulking was). The surgeon was extremely pleased and shared with my husband how fortunate I was. "One in a hundred," he said. I then had three more rounds of chemotherapy.

During all this time of treatment, my church, friends, neighbors, family, cancer survivors, support group members, and countless people I don't even know have been faithful to pray and encourage me in many ways. One day a friend sent me a note of encouragement and included the following quote from Psalm 94:19: "When doubts fill my mind, when my heart is in turmoil, quiet me and give me renewed hope and cheer." What a blessing. Because of the turmoil of my mind I often prayed for "clarity and peace of mind." During my diagnosis and treatment I was trying to be there for a dear friend who had no family. With a few other friends, we were trying to be there for her during her battle with cancer.

I have learned many things on this journey. One thing in particular is there is no coping formula that fits everyone. Some of us may stay as active as we possibly can to feel normal, while there are times that doing nothing is the perfect solution. Family and friends may tell you that you are doing too much. Listen to their counsel, but do what you must to help maintain a positive attitude. They aren't walking in your shoes. I crammed many days with things I felt I had to do, and when I made it to my front door, it was all I could do to get to the sofa and collapse. Some of us feel the need to take advantage of some complementary nutrition, treatment, and therapies. If it doesn't interfere with your treatment, only you can say if it is right for you. Tai chi has helped me with balance problems caused by neuropathy.

Years earlier in my life I found a need to remind myself daily how good the Lord had been to me and how grateful I was for His tender loving care. I realized there had been countless blessings I had received. I would thank God at the time but then almost forget the event had ever happened. I started recording at least five things a day that I was truly grateful for. This journal became quite a blessing during this new challenge in my life. It made me take note that I still had much to be grateful for: the lab technician who got the vein on the first try, the chemo nurse who helped me handle each new side effect, the soft bed I had to lie on, the doctor and his caring words and thoughtful encouragement, the Lord using those He had gifted with special talents and abilities to minister to His children in need. One journal entry says, "Am so grateful for the many people who have sent me cards and are praying for me. Lord, thank you for these brothers and sisters in Christ who are bringing my need of healing before You." What a blessing. Another entry: "God, please bless those who pray for me, and may they see Your mighty hand at work in their lives."

Earlier in my life, I had made a vow to the Lord that I would spend at least 5 minutes in His word each day. There were days my husband read to me from the Bible because I was so weak, and he knew how important the commitment was to me. This became a very special time we continue to share. Yes, I'm grateful for another of life's experiences and for the wonderful prayer warriors that helped me face it.

Bobbie Sewall

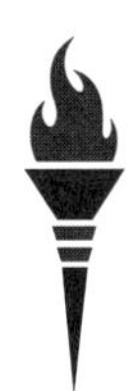

Routine Will Never Be the Same

I WENT IN for a routine vaginal hysterectomy with bladder repairs. What a surprise, when I awoke. I had stage IIIC epithelial carcinoma ovarian cancer. Dr. Michael Carley, my surgeon, called Dr. Allen Stringer, my soon-to-be oncologist. Dr. Stringer told him all the things that needed to be sent to pathology. While I was in the hospital, they did a CT scan. My new oncologist decided he would need to go back in to check for any other organ involvement. I had surgery twice in 3 weeks. Then, 24 hours out of the hospital, I was back in with a blocked colon. Five days of nothing by mouth. Two weeks later I started chemo.

My second chemo had some unusual side effects. I had a little too much Benadryl and steroids. I wanted to paint a couple of rooms, but I paced myself most of the time. With the help of drugs I used a gallon and a half of paint in one day. Of course, it took several days to get over being tired. Everyone in the family has offered to buy the Benadryl if I will come help paint their house.

After chemo they did a PET scan, and there were still cancer cells in the lymph node on my spine. They hit me with 6 weeks and 2 days of radiation. This wasn't the best time of my life, but I managed. I have not had a recurrence, so they must have done the right thing.

My children's father had a heart attack and died when they were all teenagers except the baby. She was only 6. Needless to say, my children were scared when I was diagnosed with ovarian cancer. But as we all do in a crisis, they rallied around me. They all decided on the job they would do to keep me free of stress. My son and oldest daughter went with me to every chemo treatment. One daughter kept my poodles. Another ran errands when I needed a trip to the pharmacy or McDonald's. They were all at the hospital when I was having surgery or problems. How blessed I am.

My second husband and I have been married for 20 years. We both had grown children when we married. He has one daughter and two grandchildren. I, on the other hand, have three daughters and one son. I have 16 grandchildren (at last count). Yes, he was always there when I was sick, but we always let him leave before he became too stressed. However, he did become able to stay with me until they called me for chemo. That was much better than letting me out at the door for my blood work. He did fine and fed me anything I wanted. Now I can't fuss about that.

We always worry about recurrence. While I was being watchful, I noticed my little poodle kept smelling around my breast. Of course I was concerned until one day as my dog was checking me out, I found a spot of spaghetti sauce on my shirt. So much for her worrying about my health. She was much more excited about my lunch menu.

The support group in Dallas has been one of the biggest blessings in my life. Sometimes it is heartbreaking, but all of the joys of knowing such wonderful people are more important. We cheer when someone has a good report. We understand and support each other as only someone with the same fate could do. We are members of a group that none of us ever suspected we would join. It is amazing that we come together as sisters.

My husband and I are both 65 this year. I retired in October 2003, before my surgery in May 2004. (I didn't know I was sick.) We moved to our retirement home 2 years ago. We have a beautiful yard with so many beautiful trees. I love to work outside and have learned to have a green thumb. This is a quiet place just out of Mineola, Texas. It is a very restful area. We think it is the perfect place to watch the birds (and squirrels) enjoy our bird feeders.

In my young years I was a foster parent. I have had 65 foster children. Most were infants. They always left with pictures of special days and milestones. My baby girl is one who never left. We brought her home from the hospital when she was only 4 days old. We finally adopted her when she was 15 months old, after all the legal work was finished. I love to build dollhouses when I have the time. I have one started now, but if we don't have a cold winter, I may never finish the thing. I think I will take up quilting if the winter lasts long enough.

I was the youngest child and the only girl in my family. My three brothers were a lot older than I. Need I say I have always been a tomboy? I developed a keen sense of humor. I suppose it was a survival technique.

My family was involved in a very bad auto accident 38 years ago. No one thought I had much chance of survival. However, God has given me 38 years longer than anyone ever thought I would have. I faced death head-on, and it forever changed my life. Many doors were opened for me to help when friends or family faced life-threatening crises. There have been two infants with cancer. I am so thankful for all the blessings. Most of all, I got to raise my children.

I will deal with what comes and still be more thankful for the last 38 years than I could ever grieve about the years I may lose.

Beth Robinson

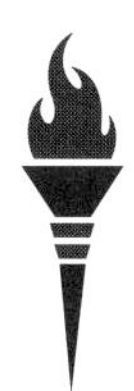

New Beginnings

IN THE SPRING of 1999, I was working very hard. I worked at an insurance company in the payroll department. I began to have severe abdominal pain. I made repeated visits to the gynecologist. There was vaginal bleeding and a lot of cramping. I was told a biopsy was not possible. My doctor did continue to prescribe hormones. A CA-125 was not done because "it was too costly." I had the symptoms of ovarian cancer but was told that I looked "too good to have it." The symptoms persisted until it was clearly time to do a D and C. The initial report: "Everything is fine."

Two weeks later I got a call saying, "The cells are changing as we speak. You need to come in." I was diagnosed with ovarian cancer that had spread to my uterus. In fact, there was a tumor the size of a grapefruit. A fibroid in the uterus was found along with an infection. During the surgery, Dr. Allen Stringer, an outstanding gynecologic oncologist, came in and completed the surgery. He said, "You can get through this." The plan was to do six chemotherapy treatments followed by a scan and then wait 3 months. I actually went every 3 months for 5 years and then was released to a gynecologist to monitor me.

I enjoyed a 7½-year remission. I was at my daughter's for Christmas in 2005. I was having a lot of abdominal pain. My primary care physician sent me back to the gynecologist for a Pap smear and an examination. A scan revealed a smooth tumor on the colon, possibly colon cancer. Surgery was done removing 3 inches of my small intestine and 3 inches of my colon. The tumor had been attached to the colon. At first, I was told that this was a different type of cancer. Yes, it was ovarian, but it had been given to me by my mother at birth, congenital. A duct had not properly shut off.

Three weeks later, I went back into Dr. Stringer. He said, "This is not a different type of ovarian cancer, June. It is the same thing." It hit me like a ton of bricks. One of the things I have appreciated most about Dr. Stringer is his ability and desire to individualize treatment. For example, I couldn't do platinum drugs because of an allergy. So, he tweaked it. When I first went in and was diagnosed, my CA-125 was 87. Now, 8 years later it is 12.

In fact, on March 1, 2007, I went in to Dr. Stringer. My treatment was finished. These are the most beautiful words you can hear after an experience like this: "You are cancer free. I see no evidence of cancer anywhere in your body. I'll see you in 3 months." You'd think I'd be dancing in the street. I have to tell you there are anxious feelings for me now. I realize I am no longer on chemotherapy. In other words, I have no safety net. There are no medications to take that would ensure the cancer would not come back.

I look back at the summer of 2000. My husband died of emphysema, my brother died of colon cancer, and my niece had inflammatory breast cancer. Grief work is hard work. I had to wrap my head around being a widow. Anger is hard work as well. I remember being so angry during this time that I yelled out at God: "Dear God, I have not done everything I want to do." I finished up my outburst by beating on the vanity in the bathroom. I actually believe I have done all that I've wanted to do.

My children live in Louisiana. They want me to move to be close to them. I have made a life here. I attend the ovarian cancer support group when I can. I have a paraplegic man living next door to me. I cook for him twice a week. Helping him actually lifts me up. It makes me feel good to know that even with cancer, I can still be helpful.

The worst part of this journey for me has been the reaction I had to the chemotherapy drugs. One of the best things about this experience is I have found out I am tougher and stronger than I thought I was. I had to reach deep inside, grab onto the toughest part, and hold on. I didn't worry so much the first time but am aware I am concerned this time. No safety net. I am a positive thinker. A positive outlook on life for me is a lifestyle. I shed negative thoughts.

One of the nicest things happened to me after I heard "cancer free." I went to the door, and there was a delivery man. He had a large, beautiful floral arrangement in his hands. "These are for you," he said. I couldn't wait to open the card to see who had sent them. My daughter, of course! The card read, "For New Beginnings." I do feel like this is a new beginning for me. It has been a long, hard struggle. I now want to enjoy my daughters and my grandchildren. I am so grateful for this opportunity I've been given. I intend to make the most of it.

June Orr

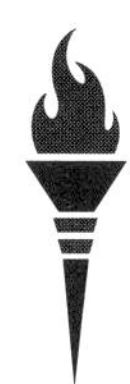

Who's in Control?
Not Me!

ORK HARD in high school—get into a good college. Do well in college—get a good job. Those were some of the lessons about achievement my parents taught me in the 1950s and 1960s when I was growing up in the Midwest. They worked for me. I did well in high school, got into a competitive women's college, graduated with honors, landed a job in the management training program of a large bank in Boston, kept my nose to the grindstone, and rose into the formerly all-male ranks of management in the bank. Later I started and ran a small landscape design business in Dallas. I managed to find a comfortable balance between work and family. I continued to believe in and practice natural consequences in other parts of my life. I believed that if you ate seven servings of fruits and vegetables daily, cut down on meat and saturated fat, took vitamin supplements, exercised 5 days a week, didn't smoke, and drank moderately, you would stay healthy. I followed the rules. I was healthy. I was in control. It worked for me—at least for 56 years, 11 months, and 15 days.

October 15, 2004, was the day I received the call from a gastroenterologist telling me that there were some "unexpected findings" on a follow-up abdominal sonogram. The radiologist suspected that I had late-stage (metastasized) ovarian cancer. That call came in on my cell phone as I was driving home from lunch with a close friend, the friend whom I had just told that I was feeling terrific. It's difficult to describe the shock that followed. Fortunately I was almost home. I drove home in a daze, heart pounding. I debated whether to call my husband, Tom, at work or just wait until he came home that evening. My rational self said "wait" and, before I even realized it, my irrational, needy self was dialing his office number. Always a man to put family first, he sensed the urgency in my voice and drove home immediately. That was the blackest day of the blackest week of our lives. Even then it was clear to us that life as we had known it had ended. There would be the life before October 15 and the life after October 15. Even though we were right, we had no way of knowing how profound the changes would be. At that point we both assumed that much of the change would be negative. From the depth of that hole it was hard to see the light that has illuminated my path, our paths, since then. It was also impossible to know how much my life and my approach to life would change. One thing was certain, though: I was no longer in control.

On October 16 I went into hyperdrive to accomplish several tasks that suddenly seemed urgent. I needed to take control of something. I called a friend who is an estate attorney; it was time to redo our wills, estate plan, powers of attorney, etc., something that had been sitting on my desk for months. In a few short days, she walked us through all sorts of difficult decisions, and we had a complete, tailor-made plan in place. Check that off the list. I started making notes about what form my memorial service should take. I made a to-do list of things I had to accomplish before I died, including organizing the photographs that are stuffed in boxes and drawers. I called a friend, a professional photographer, and asked her if she had time to come to our house and shoot some pictures of Tom and me. I didn't share with her the reason: that I knew that I would never look the same again and I wanted to record us as we looked before chemotherapy took my hair and who-knew-what-else. She unexpectedly had a cancellation for the next day and came immediately, no questions asked. I love to look at those pictures, except that I see a glimmer of terror and sadness in Tom's eyes. I managed to fake a better smile.

On the medical front, we were fortunate to have a friend and neighbor who is a prominent oncologist in Dallas. He paved the way for more tests to be done to confirm the suspected diagnosis. He got me in to see Dr. Allen Stringer, a highly respected gynecologic oncologist at Baylor Medical Center. Dr. Stringer was on vacation in New York the week of October 15, so I had to wait a week to see him. In the meantime, our friend suggested that we follow through with our plan to go to Parents' Weekend at our younger son's college.

He said that it would do us good to be distracted, since there was nothing we could do until we saw Dr. Stringer. The black veil lifted a bit as we packed and made plans to go. We called our older son in New York and asked him to join us in Providence for part of the weekend. We intended to tell both of them the news. As the weekend unfolded, we didn't find an opportune time to tell them. The restaurant where we had dinner was too small; other people could overhear. Our hotel room allowed no place for anyone to escape to process the news alone. Besides, on the television that night our beloved Red Sox, after beating the hated Yankees, were winning a World Series game. How could we spoil that? Our older son left to return to New York. Tom and I were beset with guilt about not telling the news in person. Had we abdicated our responsibility as parents? Were we such chickens? Looking back now, I realize that that was the beginning of our listening more to our hearts than our heads, something completely foreign to us achievers with fixed ideas. Maybe there really isn't one way to do things.

Also that weekend, two other important themes began to emerge. The first was the value, even the necessity, of escaping from reality. Tom and I had been socialized and educated to face things directly, not to sugar coat things, to discover the problem, face it head on, and then figure out how to solve it. Well, solving this problem was beyond us. We were in uncharted territory. And it felt so good to pretend that nothing had changed, that we hadn't heard those dreaded words. At that Parents' Weekend, no one else knew what we were fac-ing. It felt good to forget. We were stepping over the threshold into virtual la-la land for the first time, and we liked what we saw. We could laugh. Sometimes we could even forget.

The second theme we began to discover that weekend was that I want-ed—no, needed—to be near the ocean. At the time my mother died, almost 15 years earlier, I had walked the beach near her home in northern Florida. I found comfort and solace in the rhythm of the waves and the amniotic salti-ness of the water. Now that I faced a life-threatening illness, it was the place that I would find universal truths and comfort, a place that seemed eternal, a place that God and nature embraced me. We followed that theme to its logi-cal conclusion 18 months later when we bought a little house by the ocean in New England. Buying that house had been on our "list of things to do in the future," but it suddenly seemed crucial. It's La-La Land headquarters, the place where cancer is a stranger. What a gift that escape is.

The next chapter started when we saw Dr. Stringer and got a more complete explanation of the test findings and the treatment plan. The clouds began to lift; someone was in charge. It wasn't us, but we did have a plan. Calling our boys on the telephone to share the news seemed less difficult because we could also share the plan that Dr. Stringer laid out: three rounds of Taxol/carboplatin to shrink the tumors, debulking surgery, then three to five more rounds of chemo. Our inner voices, the ones we questioned, had been right. Even though we had to tell them long-distance, we could genuinely put a more positive spin on the news. There was hope, and we were going to do everything medically possible to get rid of this cancer.

After a successful debulking surgery and eight rounds of carbo/Taxol, I went into remission, my CA-125 steady at 8. Dr. Stringer explained what I knew already from my reading: the odds were very high that the cancer would recur. I wish now that I had enjoyed my 8-month remission more. Unless you've been there, it's difficult to explain that not being treated is more difficult psychologically than having chemotherapy. The specter of recurrence was like an axe over my head, and there weren't any drugs patrolling the front lines. I was just waiting for the axe to fall. And fall it did, on January 15, 2006, when my CA-125 was measured at 250. More alarming was the fact that a second CA-125 test the next day showed a 25-point jump—in just 1 day!

Recurrence—another dreaded word. But the terrible blackness didn't descend on us this time. We were more prepared for this news. Dr. Stringer pulled out all the stops and treated me with gemcitabine and cisplatin for 7 months. My CA-125 dropped steadily, but my bone marrow took a serious hit. My chemo had to be postponed multiple times because my neutrophils were dangerously low. A few times my platelets dropped too low, too. I found the emotional whipsaw of concern about low counts, multiple postponements of chemotherapy, and rescheduling my still-busy life very difficult. My life was so out of my control that I didn't know what was going to happen from day to day. For a Type A person who likes a schedule, that was a tough time.

When my CA-125 leveled off, we tried Doxil for 3 months, but it never worked at all. Suddenly we were running out of treatment options. I had been heavily treated and was platinum-resistant, and we had to regroup. As he had done all along, generous Dr. Stringer called on me to be part of the treatment team. He said that he wanted to research some options and suggested that I do the same. We would meet again in a week and share our findings.

Talk about hyperdrive—I worked at warp speed. I called some friends-of-friends with ovarian cancer to solicit their suggestions. I telephoned a couple of gynecologic oncologists in other parts of the country to pick their brains. I surfed the Internet for clinical trials and papers on treatment of recurrent ovarian cancer. Armed with a mound of printouts and notes, we met again with Dr. Stringer. I had found a protocol that was being studied in clinical trials and separate studies, and it seemed promising. In the maze of information I had unearthed, it seemed to stand out as a possibility. I can't say exactly why, but it was as if it had a little extra light shining on the page. Ironically, Dr. Stringer knew one of the researchers studying Avastin and Taxol and called him. He urged us to try it off-label, since I didn't qualify for a clinical trial. So far this combination of drugs has brought my CA-125 down from 418 to 43. I can tell that the cancer is in retreat—little "twinges" around my liver and bladder have gone away. The CT scans show that some of my diseased lymph nodes are shrinking.

I have lost the illusion of being in control, that if you're a "good girl" you'll stay healthy, and that life is fair. But I haven't lost the benefit of some of the early mechanisms I used to stay healthy and to achieve in academics and career. My educational and professional training couldn't prevent the cancer, but my ability to research a problem became invaluable as I waded through reams of treatment options, clinical trial results, etc. I tend to be insatiable when I go into research mode, losing track of time, so I do it in fits and starts as my situation changes.

I have made peace with having cancer in my body, a concept that was completely inconceivable to me BOC (before ovarian cancer). We can coexist as long as it's not growing or impinging on any vital organs. It was my yoga teacher who urged me at the very beginning to banish any warlike or aggressive metaphors from my speech and thoughts. He urged me to "welcome wellness" rather than wage a battle. I have learned to visualize my beloved ocean waves cleansing my abdomen, filling it with a healthy glow and carrying away the languishing cancer cells. In welcoming wellness, I have embraced and benefited enormously from acupuncture, Chinese medicine, and homeopathy. Acupuncture has kept the nausea under control (or gotten rid of it completely) and enhanced the energy flow through my body. I have practiced visualizations, meditation, and Qi Gong in addition to yoga. I believe strongly that there is a vital link between the mind, the spirit, and the body and that we can harness healing energies for ourselves. But, being more active than sedentary by nature, I still struggle every day to wall off the quiet time that all these activities require.

I couldn't control the fact that my immune system missed destroying that first cancer cell, but I can help my body cope with the cancer and the treatments. I believe that my well-balanced, veggie-rich diet and regular exercise have helped me weather the assault of the chemo drugs. I have continued my exercise routine religiously: low-impact aerobics, weights, and core work on Mondays, Wednesdays, and Fridays and yoga on Tuesdays and Thursdays. There have been days when I operated on sheer determination, when I had little energy and enthusiasm for moving. But I believe that the oxygenation and heat generated by regular exercise have helped keep the cancer in control and have given me a near-normal amount of energy. In addition, the endorphins produced in exercising have helped keep me depression-free and optimistic most of the time.

Fortunately, I have been blessed with a strong body, lots of energy, and a generally upbeat attitude. During this journey the past 2½ years, all those reserves have been tested, but I have been blessed to be able to maintain a fairly normal lifestyle. I appreciate the gift of each day like never before. I can't wait to turn 60, a birthday I wasn't sure I'd ever see. I smile more than ever and love life. But that doesn't mean that I haven't had dark days. The first week after diagnosis was a tear-soaked hell. Last October was difficult because my basket of chemotherapy options had emptied out. It's very scary to think that there's no treatment in reserve in case the current one stops working. I've made peace with the concept that I may be in chemotherapy the rest of my life—I'm at 39 infusions and counting. I can do this, and cancer can't take away my spirit. I can't say that I'm glad I got cancer, but I am constantly aware of all the blessings that have been showered upon me because of it.

When one gives up trying to control everything, other things are able to come into focus—"angels," for instance. Looking back on the last 2½ years, I am awestruck by the way friends and strangers drew near, offering gifts that

I didn't even know I needed. There was the yoga teacher offering his gentle wisdom about the body dealing with disease. There was a PhD candidate in psychology who, with Dr. Stringer, was conducting research on the value of individual counseling for newly diagnosed ovarian cancer patients. She held my hand for a very difficult 8 weeks. There was Dr. Stringer, who encourages hope, hugs his patients, and works tirelessly, creatively, and sensitively to help his patients. There was my sister, who dropped everything 2,000 miles away to be at my side after surgery. There was the friend who organized a large group of my friends to pray for my recovery and lay their hands on me at a weekly healing service. Tom and I have drawn spiritual and physical strength from that service every week for almost 3 years. There was the female Episcopal priest with whom I felt an instant rapport and whose generosity of spirit and faith lit Tom's and my lives, as well as those of the friends and family supporting us. There was my "mentor," a 9-year survivor of ovarian cancer and another member of our support group, who guided me through the quagmire of that first year after diagnosis. Her wisdom about protecting oneself from well-meaning intrusions and her candor about her journey and feelings have continued to help me navigate my path. There is my ovarian cancer support group, which is full of courageous women sharing and giving and holding each other close. There is my friend from college who seems to know intuitively the right thing to do and has made it clear by her words and deeds that she is there for me every step of the way. There are innumerable friends who have driven me to chemo and brought countless meals. There are friends who distract me almost daily with trips and movies, lunches and dinners. Our two boys have been more attentive than usual, yet, as I've requested, continue to lead their own lives. I know we all appreciate our holidays and vacations together more than ever. And there is Tom, my soul mate of nearly 35 years, who has been my anchor, my love, my chef, my chauffeur, my confidant, and my unfailing supporter through the dark days and the bright ones. He is unselfish and generous and optimistic. On chemo days he brings me a big bunch of roses he handpicks himself in the florist's cooler. When I have no hair, he tells me how beautifully shaped my head is. Or, when I look in the mirror and see an older woman with gray hair (well, wisps!) and new wrinkles, he swears that I've never looked more beautiful. Ah, la-la land…it's a wonderful place.

Jan Mercer

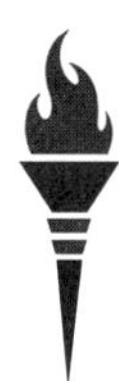

A Silver Lining

TODAY I am 40 years old. I have been married to a remarkable man for 15 years. I have two beautiful daughters, 29 and 25, since I was fortunate to marry a man with girls. My youngest daughter made me a grandmother at 35. My grandson is now 5 years old; he is my inspiration. I see myself as an adventurous professional woman, having worked in management for J.C. Penney for the last 25 years. My family and I have moved 10 times with the J.C. Penney Co., so I would say we all enjoy adventures. I was born and raised in California and currently have my home in Texas. I have a wonderful family and one sister. I enjoy my family and the time we spend together. We run/walk/yoga/ski and enjoy movies and reading.

I was 38 years old when diagnosed with ovarian cancer. Cancer does not run in my family. I had simple signs of bloating, gas, and restless nights, but this all seemed normal for my schedule. I did think I was pregnant. My husband and I were not practicing birth control, but all tests were negative. I began seeing the doctor about these symptoms in June 2004, as my symptoms had started Memorial Day weekend. June was filled with routine exams and tests like blood work, EKGs, stress tests, and x-rays—all of which were normal. Meanwhile, I could explain all my symptoms, but my friends thought I was run down. I was busy with work, and my husband kept on me to see a doctor. My doctor felt I had high blood pressure (which was borderline). This gave me relief, as I thought the doctor finally knew what was wrong with me. I started taking medication for high blood pressure in late July. I appeared to get some relief. Sometimes the symptoms of discomfort and bloating would last only one day, returning to normal the next.

After 2 weeks on medication, I began to gain weight. I called the doctor and was weighed. The comment from the doctor was "this is strange and not normal." However, my blood pressure had returned to normal. I was instructed to stop taking the medication. Meanwhile, I had a trip to California. It took everything I had to continue this trip, as the symptoms had returned. When I got back, I called the doctor right away. I was told there was nothing they could do for me, but they recommended that I go see a gastroenterologist. I was very frustrated and made an appointment, which was 3 weeks out.

On Friday I was to have my yearly visit with my OB that I almost canceled due to bloating and discomfort. When I arrived to my appointment with my OB, I began to explain what I had been going through for 3 months. She appeared to be frustrated that I was on all this medication. Once she examined me, she had difficulty finding my right ovary. She wanted me to stop all medication, including vitamins, and come back on Monday for an ultrasound. On Monday, September 14th, an ultrasound was completed in her office, and I was asked to wait for the doctor. Once my doctor arrived, she asked for my husband's number. She called my husband and began to tell us her findings once he arrived. My OB had already made my appointment with the gynecologic oncologist for Wednesday the 16th.

On Wednesday the 16th we met with my hero! My gynecologic oncologist gave us great hope. I was examined with my husband in the room, and blood was drawn. We went home to wait for results. We were called later that day, which started a whirlwind of things. My CA-125 was 2973…cancer. By Friday, September 18th, I was no longer able to walk; the fluid in my stomach made me look like I was 7 months pregnant. I was miserable. My daughter took me to the emergency room to get prepped for surgery. It was scheduled for Monday, the 20th. I did not make it through testing, so I was admitted to the hospital. I was given relief for one day when the fluid was drained off my stomach.

After surgery I was in my own room, and my doctor entered. He said if there is a silver lining to cancer, I was just given it. I had three tumors: one the size of a loaf of bread, one the size of a grapefruit, and the third the size of a volleyball. These tumors were self-contained on my right ovary. At this time he explained what was to follow: standard chemo and blood work. He also suggested I look into the opportunity of going to M. D. Anderson for a bone marrow transplant. I replied, "road trip." Today I am still astonished at my enthusiasm for the adventure.

I did make it to M. D. Anderson for the transplant. I feel very lucky to have participated in it. Today I am in remission, which did not come easy. I am truly blessed to be on this adventure and to have come this far.

Christina Huston

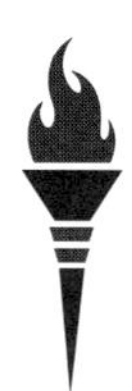

Chances Are You Remember

CHANCES ARE you can remember, with great detail, where you were when you got the word of the attack at the World Trade Center. When sitting with the memory, you can feel again some of the emotions of that September 11th morning. Horror, disbelief, fear gripped each of us.

For every woman with ovarian cancer, there is her own individual September 11th, when everything in her life changed. My September 11th was December 23, 1998. As though it were yesterday, I remember sitting in Dr. Stringer's office, frozen in fear. It was not until I walked into our house that the dam broke. I fell into my daughter's arms. She had been awaiting word. Now we began to wail. My husband took her sons down to his office to explain what was happening.

I'm happy to report that I no longer wail!

For me, nothing can duplicate the overwhelming feelings of the first diagnosis. It is as though you've been dropped in the midst of a foreign land lacking the basic vocabulary. CA-125. What's that? Next there are the relatives and friends to call and prepare to receive their various reactions. I said that I no longer wailed, but I surely did cry a lot. Fortunately, I had retired, so I had fewer commitments to cancel. I audited a course on the campus where I had taught. Having the familiarity of that space was very comforting.

People stepped in, offering help right from the start. I learned to accept the offering even though it was not what I would have requested. One of my daughters-in-law decided that, in order to keep my spirits up, I needed good make-up. It is important to know that I grew up with the following expression: It will never be noticed on a galloping horse. This translated thusly: Don't waste time preening. The consultation turned into a long, drawn-out affair. The consultant asked what I used to clean my face. I said the last bar of soap I brought home from the B & B where I had stayed. She nearly fainted, and her mission took on certain urgency. We left with my copious notes in hand determined to follow the precise order of application, fearing that a misstep could hasten disaster. Well, I have to admit that I enjoy the results of good make-up.

I learned that it was also important to initiate what I needed for my health. As Dr. Stringer finally got through to me that I would lose my hair, I decided to take control. I was running out of opportunities to exercise control in any way. I could imagine standing in the check-out line at the grocery store looking in the cart and seeing something strange. On closer examination I would identify it as my hair. So, I invited some women to come and cut my hair. We took turns, starting with me. I took a strand of hair, pulled it up, and said, "Cancer can have my hair, but it cannot have my humor." Each woman came to cut with a similar determined statement. I left the gathering empowered. My poor husband had to shave the residue. I mourned the loss of my blond hair. My husband assured me that once a blond, always a blond.

The first protocol was a bumpy ride. Plagued by low-level nausea, I never felt good. After a few weeks, my sadness wouldn't lift, and I became anxious. As the sun went down each night, I became very scared. Could I ever find myself? Would I ever be who I used to be? Fortunately, I found a wonderful psychiatrist who was a virtual Godsend. She prescribed an antidepressant and a medication to calm my anxiety. Through counseling I was able to express my scare. I began to feel more confident and hopeful. My fear that I would get overly dependent on the drugs was ill founded. As I moved into remission, I returned to the pleasures and uncertainties of ordinary life.

My husband and I determined to make hay while the sun shone. We joined a trip to Israel in which we kept up well with the group. It was substantial food for the soul. This became a prototype for how we went about planning trips. We learned to take out insurance. Sometimes we had to cancel, but more times than not, we were able to travel. Destinations included New

Zealand, a month-long trip in Europe, Ireland, Greece, Turkey, Hawaii, Italy, and a host of car trips in the U.S.

I had begun to believe that the cancer would not recur. I looked too good and felt too good. I had found acupuncture, which helped my body to detox and to keep energy flowing. I taught a Bible study. Life was familiar again. I walked at least 3 miles a day, went to Tai Chi classes, formed a monthly bridge group, joined a political action group, and worked on a political campaign. I even was hired to do some work in my profession.

I became a part of a 2-year clinical trial as I was revisiting my former life. We even took on a renovation project at our lake house, and we had lots of fun with our grandchildren. My remission had lasted 2 years, 8 months, and 5 days, but who's counting. Days elapsed in which I never even thought of cancer. So, as I went in for my usual checkup, I was stunned to find that there were changes in my CT scan. Hello, second September 11th.

Our family had been resolute in our determination to prevent cancer from moving into central command, so it was hard for all of us to absorb the blow. Our son called from California to say that he was flying in for my first chemo. I asked our associate pastor to join us in the infusion ward and to bring communion. She also brought oil of anointing, making this time with our sons, our daughter, and my husband a sacred time. When I pass through the ward, that space holds the comfort of that time. It was my habit to bring earphones and listen to a variety of music during my infusions, so this event came into a welcomed home.

I moved on to undergo three different protocols, with remissions lasting on average for 9 months. It took a while to acquaint myself with the rhythm of each regimen, but I found basically that after the first recurrence I felt listless for the first few days. I put myself under "house arrest" until some energy clicked in. I was very fortunate that my blood count was more often than not cooperating with the program. Finally, somewhere along the way it dawned on me that I have a chronic disease that I needed to manage. Now, managing the disease had more ups than downs. We flew out to California to be a part of our granddaughters' lives. We met annually with my college roommates and their husbands. It is always my best laughing time of the year. We went to North Carolina, the guests of a friend with whom I attended seminary. My stamina returned to a remarkable level. At the conclusion of this last regimen we went on a very demanding trip to Greece and Turkey. I look back in wonder.

I continued to walk faithfully, which I believe has helped keep my stamina and spirits up. I began the year with optimism and with a wonderful celebration of my 70th birthday and hoped for longer remission. I continued to volunteer at a church-operated ministry for the homeless, which gave me great satisfaction.

In the latter part of March 2006, I began to experience several odd things about my thought processes. To illustrate, it was on one of these long walks that I did something that puzzled me. I came to a curb to cross a street that would lead me to the grocery store. I stood motionless and I said, "Now what do I do?" I heard an internal voice say, "You look to the right; then you look left. If you do not see a car, then you go across the street." The symptoms became more observable to others, culminating in my unsteady walking at church where I had just taught a large Sunday school class. On the next Monday I went to get my port flushed, and my nurse, Beth, immediately saw that my reactions were delayed. The next day was my usual checkup, and Dr. Stringer saw that my talking was deliberate, as though I was working hard to get my thoughts into speech (which I was). My cancer had metastasized to my brain. September 11th made another visit. Hello, psychiatrist. It's me again.

I also had a slight recurrence of disease, but we couldn't address this issue until I concluded radiation for my brain disease. The brain cleared up after 13 treatments, and the only physical effect of the brain involvement I have is unstable walking, which does not occur every day. I am advised not to drive, and I just go about 12 blocks on back neighborhood streets to make my acupuncture appointments. My husband has been able to take me to the hospital and to take me to my sessions with my psychiatrist. Good friends have been wonderful to haul me about to other commitments.

As of this date I am still in treatment. Beating unlikely odds, it looks like I may again come to remission. We'll see.

In preparation for this article, my husband and I talked about how we had changed. Top of the list for both of us was the reordering of priorities. Just to be together seemed more critical and satisfying. We had to learn how to live with ambiguity. We still have to work on this! We like order and a predictable schedule. To a large extent, this is not possible. As we were spending more time together, we have had to define our individual interests and pursuits. It is important for each of us to have friendships and outlets. Of course, as recurrences come along, we make adjustments.

I am finding that my energy is limited, and it requires more time of rest to keep me afloat. I have to be selective with what I undertake. I hate this discipline. It is a reality that I continue to resist, but the price of fatigue is very high. I have found that fatigue leads to sadness when I come to the end of a full day with no energy left for conversations. I have coined the expression "nocturnal autism." I ask my husband to take telephone messages after 8:00 at night because I have usually shut down by then. Exceptions are our sons and daughter.

Part of the discipline of living my life is finding a delicate balance between activity that is nourishing, interesting, and downright fun and quiet time alone.

When I look at the facts of my situation, I see how remarkable these years have been. I hang on to the many words of encouragement and affirmation. When they come, it is so important to find a place in our hearts to keep the words safe so they can continue to bless us. Out of the blue our younger son called to say he was so appreciative of me for working so hard to stay alive. He said he imagined that some days I had to work harder than others, but my being alive means so much to so many. These words wash over me. Little did he know that an old friend of ours has said of me that I am relentless. Somehow this word inspires me.

Every woman must find her way through the maze of treatment. Basically, it is an invitation to trust. Trust in the goodness of friends, trust in the care that all those responsible for us extend with patience and kindness. Trust in the hope that new medications will become available. My trust in Dr. Stringer never falters. Trust that as the situation of treatment changes we will have the courage to explore, in some cases, new approaches. Trust in God's promise that we are never alone. Trust in our own wisdom about what we need. Trust that in the event of recurring September 11ths, we will find a way to go on with humor and joy.

Martha Gilmore

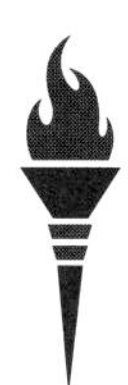

Hope, Hope, Hooray

I LOVE the picture of the Chinese philosopher who rode the donkey backwards because he liked to think of where he had been instead of seeing where he was going. It makes me smile. I don't want to live in the past, but I do believe I can learn from it. Learning is a lifetime goal of mine. Looking back, the year 2002 grabs my attention. It began with a mediation date to end a 41-year marriage. It was one of the longest days of my life. I drove home in the rain and dark. I felt as though my life would never be the same. The mediation attorney told us at the beginning, "You're not going to like what I'm going to do, but if you don't go along with it, the judge will take a hatchet to your belongings." Driving home, I didn't think the judge could have done anything that would have hurt any more than this day had. The divorce was final on February 27, 2002.

Looking back on that year, I see the spring, summer, and fall months filled with work on my dissertation, adjustment to life as a single woman, and ministry. I was doing retreats, speaking to groups of women, and looking forward to the holidays. Our Thanksgiving week was a crisis time: my granddaughter had a particularly acute asthma attack. We had four doctor visits, breathing treatments, and medications. Thankfully, she made it through. I just knew Christmas would be better. It had to be.

On Monday, December 2, 2002, I drove to the seminary to turn in my dissertation, feeling like a weight had been lifted off of me. A couple of days later, I was aware of a dull stomachache. I had a speaking engagement on Thursday, December 5, and somehow I kept it. On Friday, a nurse friend insisted I call an internist. They had just had a cancellation, and I was told to come in. My doctor examined me, shook his head, and said, "I think it's diverticulitis, but I want you to come back this afternoon for a scan." I drove home thinking, "This is awful; I'll no longer be able to eat Mexican food." I took the antibiotic he'd prescribed over the weekend and waited for his call Monday morning. I even called his office and left his nurse a message: "Call me with my report please, so I can get on with my life." I had such plans. Plans to immerse myself in ministering to women. That had been my dream. That had been my goal for 14 years of seminary. Now that I was through with school, I could get on with my plans.

My doctor did call at lunchtime. He began by saying how sorry he was. "Becky, I am so sorry, I am so surprised. It's lymphoma." I felt that I must have misunderstood. Lymphoma? He said he'd already talked with the radiologist. We needed a needle biopsy. To get into my insurance network meant I'd be going to Baylor. There isn't a day that goes by that I don't thank God for Baylor. The care I have gotten there is unsurpassed. When I was in nursing school many years ago, I'd done a rotation at Baylor. One of my first patients had advanced breast cancer. I cried all the way home that night. I had seen cancer, and it was cruel and harsh and relentless.

On December 23, 2002, my daughter and I drove to the surgical oncologist's office to get the results of the biopsy done a week earlier. "It is not lymphoma, but it is cancer. We have to figure out why your lymph system went berserk. We need to know whether it's coming from your breast, uterus, or lungs. I've already called the medical oncologist's office. Take your records to him and make an appointment." 2002 was ending with a bang: divorce, dissertation, doctorate degree, and now a diagnosis of cancer.

The appointment was made for 2 weeks later. The holidays had everyone's attention. Everyone's except mine. I went to the medical oncologist's office on January 7, 2003. He said I was a perfect candidate for an oral chemo for breast cancer. God intervened and put me with the head of the gynecologic oncology department. Thank God. Dr. Allen Stringer is the most amazing clinician and yet the most compassionate physician one could ever have on earth!!

Here it is February 2007. I'm entering my fifth year of nonstop chemotherapy. I first had carbo-Taxotere; the side effects were a bit rough, so we switched to carbo alone for almost 2 years. I remember lots of "chewing feathers" days. Then I had Taxol weekly for 11 months. I've been on Doxil for 10 months, but my doctor said he thought we had milked it for all it was worth.

My doc said, "I have been chomping at the bit to get you back on platinum." He is the captain of my ship, and I am sailing. Tomorrow I will have my first treatment of topotecan. My labs continue to be good. My recent CA-125 showed an increase from the previous month. It has been inching up for 6 months, going from 27 in September 2006 to 40 in February 2007. At my latest doctor's visit, I asked if my disease had progressed the way he had expected. "I am disappointed we didn't get to do surgery. But, I never expected you to be so durable." I have now had 100+ chemo treatments.

I had no idea how much time I would have. No one does. But, early on I made the decision not to spend whatever time I had in front of a computer doing research. I have chosen, instead, to be involved with my family, friends, and neighbors. Relationships are a priority to me. I've found they take time. Although I am a people person, I have found I need time alone. Solitude has been one of the greatest gifts. I have journaled for 27 years. It is a great comfort to me. Needless to say, I have many spirals. I hope they will one day bring comfort to my family. My journals are a record of God's faithfulness to me. He has heard and answered every prayer. Maybe not in the way I would have wanted, but His way, the best way. Whataburgers also comfort me. I screech through and laugh when the lady says, "Where have you been?" I have also built a nap into my daily routine.

Last summer when I went for chemo, I took a purple ribbon. I tied it on my chemo pole. My nurse asked, "What in the world are you doing?" We behave based on who and what we believe. I believe God had provided chemo as a way of keeping me here to accomplish His purpose. So, I said, "I am making a statement: Chemo is a gift of God to me." She kept the bow, saying others wanted to put it on their pole, too. I believe God has a plan, and cancer is not going to change it or Him. Cancer has changed me in many ways. I would not have chosen this for all the money in the world. But I would not take anything for what cancer has taught me and the incredible people I have met. God does indeed "…work all things together for good for those who love Him."

When I was diagnosed in 2003, one of the "goodest" things God did was to put in the hearts of my 35-year-old daughter and 10-year-old granddaughter the idea that they needed to move in to "take care of me." They did move in with me after a few chemo treatments. God has seen fit to put my daughter through graduate school. She is now a principal. He saw to it that my granddaughter was diagnosed and fitted for a brace for scoliosis. She wore the brace for 2 years. When it went on in 2004, my prayer was that I would be here to see it come off. It did in 2006. God has enabled me to drive myself to my doctor appointments, tests, scans, treatments. At 67, I now find myself up before the rooster crows, making breakfast, packing a school lunch, and in the carpool line. I also find myself dyeing Easter eggs, carving pumpkins, putting out cookies for Santa, planning extravagant teenage birthday parties, and buying lots of hair products though I have none. Our home is filled with the sounds of teenage girls. We even have sleepovers, though I'm not sure who came up with that name. God willing, I will baptize my granddaughter Easter 2007 in my friend's pool.

Looking back, I'm reminded that I have not and am not going to face anything that is bigger than God. All I have needed His hand has provided. He is worthy of my trust. I've also learned the enormous value of walking closely with others on this road. A support group is essential. Research proves that those in a group do better emotionally and physically. If you do not have one, start one. God will put it together, and you will be amazed at the variety, beauty, and strength of the women. Their capacity to love one another, bear burdens, encourage and inspire one another will profoundly affect the way you view life. At times, their thoughtfulness and kindness to one another will over-whelm you. Their ability to celebrate the good news and suffer when there's bad news will deeply touch your heart and soul. My circle of simply incredible sisters causes me to daily thank God for the way He has knit us together.

Ovarian cancer has marinated me in mercy. I have been tenderized. I've always been a strong, able, "doer" woman. In the past, I toted ladders, plant-ed shrubs, painted, caulked, mowed, trimmed, and wallpapered. If it needed doing, I could do it. Now, I'm learning the value of being still, listening instead of talking, giving thanks, being generous with the "I love you's," "thank you's," and "I'm sorry's." I'm so thankful for these years of time with my family and friends. I never thought I'd see five Christmases or five birthdays. I celebrate every day!

I've heard that life is understood backwards but has to be lived forward. Looking back, it has been quite a journey. Looking forward, my eyes are wide open to the possibilities. I've heard when you think of the future, you either feel fear or hope. I am a hope, hope, hooray person. In 1956, our little blonde cheerleaders taught us a yell. They told us we were all winners. We went all the way to state! That yell has stayed with me all these years. It goes like this: VI, VI, VICT… TO, TO, TORY… VICTORY, VICTORY… YEA!!!!! One of the first things Dr. Stringer told me was, "Becky, it is not hopeless." I have a great physician on earth, and I have the Great Physician in heaven. Therefore, I have endless hope. And so do you!

Becky Teter

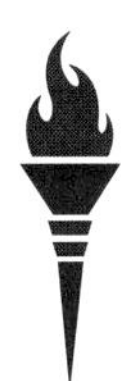

God Kept Me

THAT'S THE TITLE of my favorite song. I love the melody, the words, but more importantly the reminder it is to me, a very personal reminder. It is the hymn a young lady sang and dedicated to me my first Sunday back to church after a life-threatening, life-changing event. The surgical report read, "She almost coded. We had to bring her back." I think that would be called a defining moment. Also, a lady told me she knew I would walk back in that church.

My name is Louise Kelley. I am a 77-year-old African-American woman. The word I would use to describe myself is "blessed." I've been married for 58 years…to the same man! We have two sons, and I am blessed to be here for two granddaughters and to see my five great-grandchildren. When I think back, I can remember, as if it were yesterday, seeing my husband for the first time. I had never dated, but I surely didn't want him to know that. So, when he approached me, I made up a name. "I've been dating Anthony," I said. I didn't even know an Anthony. We dated for a year and then married.

I am the oldest of five children. My mother died when I was very young. The responsibility for my four siblings fell to me. It was a heavy load. I started caregiving at an early age. My husband says now, "God has spared you so you can take care of me." God certainly has kept me. I know it is for a purpose. My husband is not in good health and does need care. That is surely part of the purpose, but I believe there is more He wants me to do. My granddaughter is also sick, and she has three children.

I'm going back to 2003 to tell my story of ovarian cancer. It was then that I started having symptoms: low abdominal pain, bloating, and losing weight. One Sunday, the pain was so bad that I knew I needed to go to the hospital.

I checked into the emergency room on March 8, 2004. They discovered a blockage. Before then I had gone to my primary care physician. A scan found nothing; it was clear. I went to the gynecologist. She found nothing. Maybe a bladder infection, she thought. I got a prescription for an antibiotic. Another trip back to my primary care doctor who said "We don't find a thing." That appears to happen often. Other women I hear say the same thing, "We were missed, dismissed."

On March 13, 2004, I had surgery for the blockage. I'd had a colonoscopy a year earlier and it had been clear. After surgery, one doctor said, "You might as well take all that stuff/equipment off of her. She's had a heart attack. She's not going to make it." Thankfully, my pastor was standing there and offered, "No, the devil is a liar. Don't you dare take it off." Later, another doctor came and said, "She's going to make it." I was in the intensive care unit for 12 days, on a hospital floor for 5 days, and then sent to a rehab facility for 6 days. I don't remember much of the ICU experience except that someone told me to repeat The Lord's Prayer over and over. I did that. I also kept talking scripture to myself. God kept me then, and He has continued to keep me. My son said he asked me if I wanted them to take off the equipment, and I said "No." I don't remember his asking me that.

I do remember the oncologist asking me, "Do you want to do chemo?" I said, "Yes, I do." He said, "It could be a year, two, five or whatever. We never know." I went to my primary care physician, and he said I might have until December. I was diagnosed with stage IV ovarian cancer, and in everyone's opinion I didn't have very long. God obviously thought otherwise.

When I began this journey, my cancer marker was 1,500. After chemo, it went down to 34. Now, in March 2007, the marker is 10. I had a memory of a relative picking up my chart, reading it, and shaking her head in a "not good news fashion." I have gone back and asked her, "What did you read that made you shake your head?" She doesn't remember. I don't know that it really matters much now. Three years later, I am still here.

We used to travel a lot. I love to cook. Soul food is my specialty: turnip greens, sweet potatoes, okra, black-eyed peas, broccoli, cabbage, and red beans. I always have something green for dinner. I like to cook extra on Sundays in case somebody comes by. I am trying to be careful about my diet. I have cut down on sugar. Going to the grocery store is something I love to do. I am not much of a shopper, except for groceries. The ladies in my support group are always talking about my being "a snappy dresser, many accessories." One said, "Louise, you have got to be our poster woman."

I noticed about 8 months ago that the feelings of depression began. I've not been a worrier, but I do remember one time crying so hard because I was hurting. Since then, the one thing I worry about is my health. I go to the local YMCA twice a week for exercise. I think that helps me feel better. I really didn't have bad side effects from the chemotherapy drug Doxil. No nausea, no vomiting. At times depression is still with me. I've got a clear conscience. I don't think there is anything I want to say that I haven't already said. I have dealt with unforgiveness. I think when you don't forgive a person, that is self-abuse. It hurts you, not the other person. With my husband in bad health and my condition, I do know my other family members are doing all they can to take care of us. I am doing my best. *I am too blessed to be stressed.*

What would I tell someone who has just heard, "You have ovarian cancer"?

The first thing I would say to them is "Trust in God, not in man." Trusting in man would have resulted in the hospital personnel removing "all the stuff" from me. God spoke through my pastor. I made it. So, I give thanks to God, Who has kept me.

I thank the hospital and the medical staff for my care. I thank my oncologist. He says I am doing better than he thought I would.

Back to my title, "God Kept Me": the devil thought he had me, but God reached and got me. He held me close so I wouldn't let go. I am still here today by His grace.

I don't know what the future holds, but I do know Who holds the future.

Louise Kelley

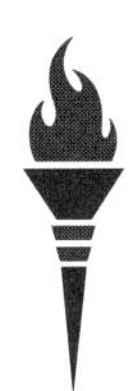

Cancer: A Monumental, Life-Changing Event

I WAS 41 years old, a full-time mommy, a full-time respiratory therapist, buying a home, moving, and busy living my life. I didn't feel sick; I didn't have time to be sick. I had acid reflux and needed to lose weight. I went to see my primary care physician for my annual checkup, a mammogram, and birth control pills. What I got was an MRI, a visit to Texas Oncology, and a hysterectomy. I also lost 10 pounds and a cantaloupe-sized ovarian tumor.

Late on July 9, 2004, I woke up from general anesthesia to see my doctor. He had tears in his eyes when he told me it was ovarian cancer and it was stage III. I was numb; I was sad; I was overwhelmed. But I knew, deep down inside. I knew after the MRI that it was cancer. I had planned on the worst-case scenario. I had cried driving to and from work, from Canton to Dallas; I had read everything on the Internet; I had done my research. But no one is really ready to accept the worst. I now had a terminal illness. I was going to die.

But in Penni fashion, I decided I would be like Scarlet O'Hara. "Why fiddle-dee-dee! I don't want to think about that right now; I will think about this tomorrow." I have always been one to have a good pity party (this time I allowed myself a couple of weeks), then wipe my eyes, blow my nose, and say, "Okay, now what am I going to do about this?" I first had to heal from my surgery. Then, I had to plan my chemotherapy. Then, it would all be over, and I could get back to my life on my terms. I had a 4-year-old daughter that needed a mommy. I needed to be in her life for all the skinned knees, broken hearts, dance recitals, report cards, graduations—every dream a mommy has for her child. I had also started working at Children's Hospital in Dallas. I was fulfilling my dreams and plans. I had found a house as big as I wanted, with 4½ acres of land; I was going to have green grass to mow, goats to play with, and maybe even a cow or a horse. This was just one of those little bumps in the road of health I would get over as quickly as a cold.

Unfortunately, life is not always as we plan. I healed from surgery; I had the first six rounds of chemo. My mom and dad came to live with us. Finances got very tight. Getting back to work was slower than I had hoped. The side effects and fatigue were physically, emotionally, and spiritually draining. Three months after round one of chemo my counts (tumor marker) were going up. I started chemo again. Every month I have chemo. It took over a year for me to finally accept that this is not going to go away. This is an ongoing chronic issue. I still live my life the way I want. I just have to schedule in my chemo, plan on the bad days, and live for the good days.

Like Scarlett O'Hara, I have determined never to give up. I have a beautiful daughter who is my light, my hope, my joy, and my reason to get up every morning even if I do not want to. I still have my career at Children's Medical Center in Dallas. They have been wonderful to me. They work around my chemo schedule and all my sick days. I have learned to slow down a bit, take time out for me and my family. My husband and I went to Alaska and brought his mom to come and live with us. We just went on our first cruise. We are now planning our summer vacation. I still don't feel sick, although fatigue is my new best friend. My cancer is still there. My counts go up and down, but I am *stable*. As long as I am stable, I am living. I take life one day at a time.

Some of my favorite sayings:

- Cancer is not for sissies.
- Cancer sucks!
- This too shall pass.
- In the spirit of Dory on *Finding Nemo*, "Just keep going. Just keep going."
- My mission for you, if you choose to accept it, is "Be Happy! Don't Worry!"
- Live every day as if it is your last.

And always say your good night prayers: "Now I lay me down to sleep, I pray thee Lord my soul to keep. If I should die before I wake, I pray thee

Lord my soul to take. If I should live another day, I pray thee Lord to guide my ways. Amen."

Penni Bourque

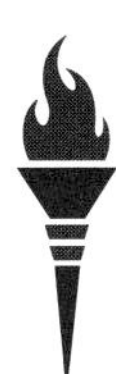

The Gift of Today

I WAS RECENTLY driving through New Mexico in very heavy fog, at night, on unfamiliar roads. My granddaughter thought it was grand, "like bumper cars, Nana. All you have to do is stay between the lines." I had to remind her that with bumper cars the object is to bounce off the bumpers of all the other cars on the track—something I hoped we would not be doing!

The fog was heavy for a long time, but as day was breaking, the fog gradually began to lift. It was sporadic and would change from foggy to clear and then back again several times before ultimately clearing altogether. When the fog lifted, the road signs were distinct and clear and very easy to read. I looked around further. The beauty of this day was just beginning, and I was taken aback in awe.

It occurred to me how similar my journey with cancer has been. Like in the fog, when I was first diagnosed, I could hardly see anything. It was black and dark. I was scared. The beams of light offered no look into the future, but rather reflected helplessly back into my immediate path. Instead of looking at the big picture, I had to concentrate on just staying between the lines.

My first CT scan showed cancer throughout my abdomen. Pancreas, ovaries, omentum, spleen, possibly colon, and liver…the list goes on. My son was with me when I got the news, but I couldn't bring myself to call my daughter. Luckily my son called her, and she drove all night to be with me. I went home and cried in my sweetheart Richard's arms. We scheduled an emergency sisters' meeting so I could tell them in person. It had to be done, but having recently lost another sister to breast cancer, it was not easy. I just knew my life would be over in 6 months or less.

Like the fog, the next few weeks were a blur. There were blood tests, biopsies, and a PET scan. On the way to my doctor's office, I pulled out a copy of the PET scan and saw the blanket of malignancy wrapped around my liver. This can't be good. Additionally, the biopsies confirmed two primary malignancies: ovarian and islet cell cancer of the pancreas.

Decisions had to be made. How do you make decisions when your life depends on it? I researched on the Internet and became even surer of my impending demise. Luckily I had the support of family and friends. They dragged me along and helped me stay on course. I also *stopped* searching the Internet. I later learned that by the time statistics are published they are already outdated.

I was also tested and found positive for the *BRCA1* gene. I officially had a 90% chance of breast cancer and a 40% chance of ovarian cancer. I also learned there were other cases of ovarian cancer in my family—a grandmother and a cousin, both of whom had died from this. Additionally, I had two sisters and a mom who had had breast cancer (twice each). My siblings were tested as well. Two were positive for the genetic mutation; two were negative. My kids were tested: one positive, one negative. I was told I would need to be in remission for 2 years before a "decision" would need to be made about my breasts. Both of my sisters who were positive, however, opted for prophylactic surgery. They found early ductal breast cancer in one. I was relieved that she would not have to go through chemo.

I opted to have my debulking surgery in the middle of the chemotherapy regime. They would also do a pancreas resection for the pancreatic cancer. (Though one physician suggested since I was stage IV, perhaps surgery was not a good option for me.) A total of eight chemos were scheduled. Luckily I responded almost immediately to chemo. Surgery was done after number four and was considered a success because they were able to "optimally debulk." I continued to work long hours and took the minimum of time off that I felt I needed. I continued to drive too fast on this fog-saturated road. Just stay on course, I told myself, and you'll get through this. I guess I thought the faster I drove, the faster I could get this behind me. During this time I did attend a support group for women with ovarian cancer. The meetings were held at Baylor University Medical Center in Dallas.

I completed that treatment regime on November 11, 2005. Still burning the candle at both ends, I went to my daughter's house to help her after her C-section scheduled for 3 days later. While there, I got high fevers and even passed out in the bathroom and broke some ribs. I saw a physician locally who administered IV antibiotics and rehydrated me.

My boss and other people at work were very supportive. My boss even suggested I take long lunches and travel to the Baylor support groups whenever possible. I was terrified, but something else was happening to me as well. I began to take less joy in my work, something that had once actually defined me. Many aspects of my job seemed very trivial. I found myself using mortality as a measuring stick for everything. This is beneficial when, for instance, you have a spat with your loved one and you just need to get over it. But, at work, even trivial things need to be addressed. I continued to do my job, but it was getting more difficult, not returning to normal like I thought it would. The fog remained heavy as I continued to work too much. I often worried about a recurrence.

The support group was wonderful. I could be myself there, and they understood. "What do I look for in a recurrence?" I asked one day. The women discussed their own experiences. They talk and share, but advice is never given, just support and understanding.

It is strange to say, but the fog started lifting after my recurrence. Not feeling I needed to be the hero anymore, I took a leave of absence from work. This time around I would take better care of myself. I am enrolled in a yoga class and go to the support group most weeks. I am in a good place most days. The fog is gone, and everything is bright and clear. It's a different life. It revolves around doctor visits and lab and radiographic tests, but it's not a bad life. It's a shame but, without this experience, I would not be at this place. For the most part I have quit worrying about my mortality. My mantra now (I heard this one day at support group from a very wise woman), "My days are numbered by the Lord, and only he knows when that time will be up and whether it will be by heart attack, accident, or ovarian cancer." There is a reason they call each day the "present."

Joyce Camp

"Faith isn't Faith until it's all you're holding on to." (Author unknown)

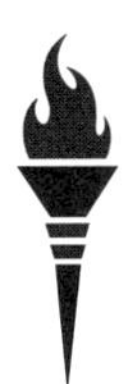

How the Worst Time Can Be the Best Time

WHEN SCOTT, our firstborn, was 6 months old, Charles and I made a commitment to serve the Lord. Even though we've fallen short way too often, God has always been faithful to us. He entrusted us with three beautiful children (Scott, Lori, and Kristy) and blessed us in many ways as we raised them. Now they were grown and caring for their own families, and it was time for us to retire, to travel, and do the things we enjoy. Or so we thought.

When I'd been retired only a few months, in mid-September 2004, the mail brought one of those postcards from my gynecologist, "time for your annual checkup." I was feeling good, finally over a bad sinus infection, so I tossed it in with my bills thinking I'd get to it soon.

Suddenly that weekend I started having a lot of uncomfortable bloating in my stomach. I told Charles, "This reflux is really acting up. It's so bad I may need that surgery I've been reading about." So Monday I retrieved the card and called, requesting an appointment for my annual physical, saying nothing about my symptoms. The receptionist asked, "Can you be here this Wednesday at 2:30?" I couldn't believe I could see the doctor that quickly; usually it took several weeks! I didn't realize it then, but that was the first indication that God would be with me in the coming ordeal.

I was going on about my symptoms when Dr. Green interrupted me. "Dot, I'm sorry to tell you this, but you have a mass. I don't know what it is, but it's big. I want you to have a blood test today and come back tomorrow for a sonogram." I guess my mind was playing tricks on me, but until then I hadn't thought about the possibility of cancer. My first reaction was fear, but it was immediately followed with what I can only describe as a picture of a ticker tape going through my mind with these words: "Yea, though I walk through the valley of the shadow of death I will not be afraid, *for thou art with me.*" I knew right away it was reassurance from the Holy Spirit, and I told my doctor, "It's in the Lord's hands." There was no assurance that I would be healed, just a certainty that He would be taking every step I did no matter what they found.

On Thursday, September 29th—Scott's 37th birthday—Dr. Green called with the results of the tests. Charles had just retired from the clinic, and Dr. Green knew him well, so they talked. Charles, hanging up with tears in his eyes and voice cracking, said, "All indications are that it's ovarian cancer."

I was stunned! Except for my paternal grandfather, who had a facial cancer back in the early 1940s, no one in my family had cancer (at least not to my knowledge). The only lady I had known to have ovarian cancer died from it at the age of 49. So I thought I had been given a death sentence. How can I describe the thoughts and fears whirling through my mind? I wanted to run so far I would outrun it. I wanted to scream and turn back the clock about 4 days. I was afraid I couldn't handle it, that I would be a wimp. All these thoughts and more flashed through my mind while Charles was telling me what the doctor said. I stood there facing him, trying to listen over the roaring in my ears, and I prayed, "Lord, you know my makeup. On my own I will be a basket case. Please give me your strength and help me handle this. I want to be strong." Before I could even say "Amen," warmth flooded through me, from the top of my head to the ends of my fingers and toes. It was God's peace and a sense of His love for me, and it stayed with me throughout the ordeal. I've spent most of my life fighting feelings of inferiority and negativism, but contrary to what you would expect, I had a radical change in my thinking. I became a much more positive person. I felt totally accepted and overwhelmingly loved—by God, by other people, and even by myself.

"Think about going to M. D. Anderson," Dr. Green suggested. "If your insurance doesn't pay for chemotherapy, Anderson will work with you. The doctor who wrote the book on ovarian cancer is there; however, he trained the oncologists at Baylor." But our very supportive older daughter, Lori, lives in

Plano with her family, and we are only an hour away, so we decided to stick with Baylor.

When we called the number my doctor gave us for the appointment, we were told to be there in 2 weeks. "My wife is very uncomfortable. Can't you get her in any sooner?" Charles asked. "Tell her if she's that uncomfortable to go to the emergency room! We are booked solid, but if we get a cancellation, we will call you," was their seemingly uncaring retort.

At home we waited, uncomfortably, for the oncologist appointment. One day we were out running errands. When we returned home at 1:15 p.m., there was a message on the answering machine from Baylor. "We had a cancellation, and we can work you in if you can be here at 1:30 p.m. today." Of course we couldn't make it in 15 minutes!

That turned out to be another way God was watching out for my best interest, because the very next day we received a call from Texas Oncology, a group of gynecologic oncology doctors who also have offices at Baylor Hospital. I don't know how they got my name, but the lady said, "The place where you have an appointment is the free clinic. Do you have insurance that will pay for chemotherapy?" I answered, "They say they will. Here's the name and number if you would like to call and verify it." Within 30 minutes she called back and affirmed what my booklet said. They worked me in the next business day (which was a Monday). Somehow my local doctor had it in his mind that my insurance would not pay for chemo. Right or wrong, it seems that you get better care if you have insurance. I strongly believe that God had His hand in it and He was directing me to Dr. Allen Stringer, a wonderfully capable and compassionate Christian gynecologic oncologist.

I wanted to take all the steps I was supposed to and be certain that I had all the t's crossed and i's dotted just right, so I followed the advice in James 5:13–15: "Is any one of you sick? He should call the elders of the church to pray over him and anoint him with oil in the name of the Lord. And the prayer offered in faith will make the sick person well; the Lord will raise him up." I discussed it with my pastor, Rev. Tony Neal. One Wednesday night after the service, Rev. Neal and three of his deacons came to my house, anointed me with oil, and laid hands on my head and prayed for me, even though they emphasized that we should pray for God's will more than my physical healing. Well, I believed that, and I knew for certain that God had touched me and He would indeed work out His will for me (even without these steps), but I was doing everything I knew to do. I didn't want to leave any stone unturned!

During the second week after my diagnosis, I started gaining weight—rapidly. I gained about 20 pounds from the time of my original diagnosis to the day of my surgery 3 weeks later. As if I had a huge balloon inside, my tummy was also protruding by leaps and bounds. I soon looked like I was about to deliver a baby. When Dr. Stringer examined me on October 12, 2004, I could tell a significant difference in the examination from when Dr. Green examined me 2 weeks before. "This tumor has spread, and I don't know if we can do surgery now. We may have to start with a couple of chemo treatments to shrink it first," Dr. Stringer told me. "Chemotherapy is effective about 80% of the time. But I will schedule you for a CT scan tomorrow, and we'll make that determination after we see the results," he added.

That night I went to the ladies' Bible study at church. About 25 to 30 women have been meeting regularly for about the last 8 years, and we have grown a lot through our studies. I told the ladies the events of the day. "Please pray that the chemotherapy is effective," I requested.

The next day Charles was driving me to Baylor, and about the time we went through Ennis I told him, "I don't know how to explain it, but something is happening to my body." For lack of a better way to describe it, it was like tiny, almost not there flutterings, but not really. Perhaps it was more of a sensation, or maybe just a whisper of knowledge, but I was convinced God was doing something! Since my appointment wasn't until 6:00 p.m., it wasn't until mid-morning the next day, Wednesday, when the doctor called. "Good news, Dot, the CAT scan indicates we can indeed proceed with the surgery next week." I will always believe it was the prayer from the ladies of my church that made the difference!

Dr. Jonathan Oh, my surgeon, set the time for 11:30 a.m. on October 19th. My family and several dear friends started arriving about 9:00 a.m. The ladies in our Bible study group sent word that at 11:30 they would stop what they were doing, get down on their knees, and pray for my successful surgery.

I didn't know all of this until much later, but the surgery lasted 5½ hours. "We removed four tumors, and the largest was the size of a soccer ball. We also removed her ovaries, the omentum, and parts of each of the large and small intestines." Dr. Oh went on to tell them, "We know there are two tumors that were too small to be removed, and her chest has so many precancerous cells it looks like someone threw a cup of rice at her. We could have gotten it all, but it would have taken 19 hours, and she would not have been able to hold up to it."

The surgery was on a Tuesday, and they kept me in the ICU until Friday, explaining there were no rooms available on the ovarian cancer ward. I was sedated most of that time, but I do remember snatches of family coming to see me. One memory that stands out is of Scott waving an angel figurine that he had purchased and kept right over my bed, assuring me that angels were watching over me.

Once they admitted me to a private room, I made rapid progress. Dr. Oh discharged me on Wednesday, 8 days after the surgery, stating, "I'm surprised at how well you are doing." Anytime he made a comment on that order, I would quickly assure him it was because many people were praying for me. I was 35 pounds lighter when I left the hospital than I was before my surgery.

Prior to the first treatment, my doctor gave me samples of an antinausea drug named Emmend. The next evening I got just a bit sick to my stomach, but throughout the 6 months of treatments, I never again experienced nausea nor did I ever vomit. My problem was weakness, dizziness, and shortness of breath. If I cooked, I had to keep a chair near the stove and counter because I could not stand for any period of time. I was so forgetful it was embarrassing! When I told Dr. Stringer how weak and dizzy I was after the first treatment, he assured me it was only to be expected. "After all, you had a traumatic surgery that you weren't healed from by any means, followed by the chemo in only 2½ weeks. So you had a double whammy!"

Dr. Stringer warned me that I would lose my hair, and just about everyone whom I talked with agreed. Karla, a friend who lived in our community and is a member of our church, had been my beautician for several years. I phoned her, "Karla, everyone tells me I'm going to lose my hair. If it happens, I want to come in and let you shave it, but I don't want to do it in front of your mirror where I can see what's happening. I would like for you to do it in your back room. Then I will don one of my hats and go home to my bathroom where I can scream as loud as I want to."

Several days after the first treatment, my head was sore for a few days, but I didn't shed any hair! After all, I reasoned, the Bible says a woman's hair is her glory, and maybe this is another way the Good Lord is blessing me. When I returned for my next appointment, I proudly told everyone that I still had my hair, but Dr. Stringer deflated me. "Your hair will most assuredly fall out." On day 17 after the second chemo, my hair began to shed. For 3 days it was in everything—even my mouth. So I called Karla and told her it was time.

She was an angel. "You don't need to be out in this cold, wet weather. I will come to your house in the morning before I go to work," she insisted. When she arrived, I was crying. Throughout the diagnosis, the surgery, and the first two chemos I remained dry-eyed and upbeat; I suppose it's silly to get so hung up about something that's so minor in relationship to everything else, but the thought of losing my hair was devastating. "Dot, I can just cut it short; then if you see the need, I can come back later. We don't have to shave it today!" she offered. But her husband, Bubba, was facing major surgery the following week, and I didn't want to bother her to return for the second time (especially when she wouldn't let me pay her!). "This is a talent the Lord gave me, and I want to do it for you," she insisted. So out came the razor, and down went my hair!

That's just an example of how wonderful and kind people were to me during that time. Charles stuck to me like glue and did everything I couldn't. My children were very loving and supportive. When I was diagnosed, I told a few friends, and before long I found out I was on the prayer list of many individuals and churches throughout the whole United States. People brought food, called and sent cards, and showed me God's love in many ways. My church even gave me a hat shower! Liz, one of my best friends, called me every day for 6 months, even when she was out of town. I also met a few of the ladies from the support group at Baylor who will never know what an inspiration they've been to me.

But I absolutely hated looking at myself in the mirror. I was always careful to have my head covered with a hat or a wig (I had two). After a few months I started wearing a baseball cap around the house; finally I loosened up enough to go "bald" when only Charles and I were there. One day as we sat down to eat lunch, I asked him, "Charles, does it bother you or put you off for me to come to the table with my head bare?" I was so touched by his response, "Not at all. When I see your head, it reminds me of how good God has been to us."

While I was having my sixth chemo treatment, Beth (Dr. Stringer's nurse) handed me a card with the dates and times of my next appointments. "You will have the CAT scan, then a week later an appointment with Dr. Stringer, but…he said it is not necessary to schedule any further chemotherapy." The feeling of relief mixed with gratitude was simply overwhelming!

At home I resolved to get back to my routine as quickly as possible, walking just a bit more each day, resuming household chores, thanking God for each new day when I awoke. I testified to God's goodness and mercy at every opportunity. But the closer it got to the next 90-day checkup, the more anxious I became. The fear of it returning is said to be worse on cancer patients than the treatment, and I found out what that meant. "What if it comes back? What if it comes back?" was a constant refrain that would not turn me loose. I prayed and asked God for help, and He never failed to calm me. But it wouldn't be long until I once again was on the brink of a panic attack. I was grumpy, lashing out at my husband (and others) when they didn't deserve it, and I was eating everything in sight. Finally I got desperate and prayed, "Lord, you know my heart, and you know I *do* trust you. You have proven yourself to me over and over, and I don't know why I am so anxious about this. Please take this fear away from me *once and for all.* You know I don't want to live like this!"

That night a lady about my age knocked on our door. She introduced herself as a friend of my neighbor and inquired, "What kind of cancer was it?" When I said ovarian, she nonchalantly replied, "Oh, I had that in 1989. The doctors kept close tabs on me for a while, but then my checkups got further apart until finally they said to resume my regular, annual checkups. I've been fine ever since." Well, she was attractive and looked quite healthy, so I took that to be the answer to my prayer. I was finally able to settle down. Sure enough, when I had all the tests in June, the doctor came in with a big smile and the welcoming words, "All is well. We don't detect any signs of cancer." As of this writing it's been nearly 2½ years since my surgery and 2 years since my last chemo treatment, and so far, that's the same report I get every time.

Our younger daughter, Kristy, was 33 when she found out she was expecting her first baby. We already had four precious grandchildren, but I had no assurance that I would live to see the baby of our baby, who was due in March 2005. One day while I was reading, these words jumped out at me: "May you live to see your children's children" (Psalm 128:6). I claimed that verse, and the day I had my fifth chemo treatment that lasted for 5 hours, Kristy had her baby. We left Baylor Hospital in Dallas at 6:00 p.m. and had been in the hospital room in Round Rock about 10 minutes when they brought Tyler to his mother for the first time! As of this writing, we have just returned from going to his second birthday party! Every time I look into Tyler's beautiful eyes I think about God's love and His wonderful promise to me.

My husband said I have a glow about me, like I've faced the giant and won. That I have, although I don't think for one minute that I should get credit for any of it. Actually, it is more of an awe over what God has done for me through all this. It was the Lord, pure and simple, that gave me peace and strength and His healing touch. Yes, I had faith, but the Bible tells us that even our faith is a gift from God. So the fact that I can sit here and write this—cancer free—is only because of His love and grace.

So you see this story is not really about me. It is mind-boggling to me that the God who rules the universe and has billions of people to care for knew all about my troubles and cared enough to answer my prayer before I even said "Amen." I've asked Him why He blessed me so and what I'm supposed to do about it now. One day when I was reading the Bible these words from Psalm 118 jumped out at me, "You will live and not die and will proclaim what the Lord has done." Whether I live one more year or thirty, this is what I am attempting to do. I have no real assurance that there won't be a recurrence (although several people told me they prayed that I would be healed and that "it will never return again"). If it should, I'm aware that the outcome could be entirely different. There's only one thing I am certain of. I have the strength and peace that only He can give. I can handle anything that happens to this old body.

I believe He has used me through this to be an instrument to show others His love and power and to offer hope and encouragement no matter what your circumstances are. There are different kinds of healing, and it's not always physical, but for everyone whose heart is right with God and turns to Him for help, His word promises that He will be our refuge and strength and an ever-present help in times of trouble (Psalm 46:1). I thank Him every day for His presence and for the way He understands me, relieves all my anxieties, and provides just what I need for every situation (read Philippians 4:6–7).

The paradox is that while I hope and pray with all my heart it never returns, in many ways my experience during those dark days is the best thing that ever happened to me. My prayer is that everyone will experience the reality of our awesome God in her own life.

Dot Reynolds

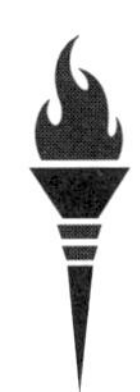

Life Is Like a Box of Chocolates

IT WAS August 2000 and a hot summer in Texas when I decided to cool off by visiting my best friend, Carol, in Vermont. One of the activities she had planned for us was to climb a small peak called Bald Knob, which is part of the White Mountains. I am not a very athletic person, but I figured I could easily climb this. I had not gone very far when I had to stop. I huffed and puffed and could only go about 20 feet without stopping to rest. I did make it to the top of the peak but was exhausted and felt like I had climbed Mt. Everest.

After returning to Dallas and my office job, I took stock of the symptoms I had been having. My energy level was lower than I had ever felt it; just getting out of bed in the morning was an ordeal. I had a pain in my left side. However, the most alarming thing was my belly seemed to be growing daily, almost as if I were pregnant. Well, I was 50 years old, had a hysterectomy in 1993, except my ovaries were not removed, and there was no way I was pregnant. I was not gaining weight, but none of my pants fit. I had to keep the button unbuttoned, and in some cases even keep the zipper down a ways.

I already had an appointment in late September with my gynecologist, so I figured I would wait and tell her about my symptoms. So I suffered through another month before seeing a doctor about my problems. When I did see her, she chalked it up to a bladder infection, gave me a prescription for an antibiotic, told me to call her in 3 weeks if it didn't get better, and sent me on my way.

Several weeks went by, and my symptoms only got worse. By late October I looked like I was about 7 months pregnant, and I was getting very worried. Rather than return to my gynecologist, who was young and treated mostly soccer moms, I went to my internist of 20 years. He was in his 60s, and I just felt more comfortable with him since his patient base was mostly middle-aged. Why I didn't go to him in the first place, I really don't know. My mistake. He seemed concerned about the symptoms, gave me an exam, and set up an appointment for a sonogram, and, if necessary, a CT scan.

It was October 31, 2000, and I had left work to go get the tests done, thinking I could return to work in the late afternoon, finish up a few things, and then head to my son's house to watch my precious granddaughter, 2 years old, go out for her first Halloween of trick or treating. I did the sonogram, then the CT scan. The technician came out and said sweetly, "You need to go over to your doctor's office. He would like to talk to you." Somehow I got an ominous feeling. There I sat in the examining room with my pumpkin vest on, waiting for my doctor, when he opened the door with a quite dour look on his face. He said, "There is no good way to tell you this. You have advanced ovarian cancer." I never put that vest on again and never went back to work except to clean out my desk.

I am a big movie buff, and I have seen many a movie where a character is told, "You have cancer." It always seems so sad and dramatic, the music swells, and I get tears in my eyes. When it happens to you in real life, there are just not words strong enough to convey how devastating it is to hear that.

From that point, my internist quickly made a phone call and referred me to a female gynecologist/oncologist at Baylor Hospital. He said, "She's the best; she will take care of you." Two days later my husband and I were sitting in her office. It was late in the afternoon on a Thursday. She said, "You have stage IIIC ovarian cancer. You will need surgery as soon as possible and also chemotherapy." She said she had a surgery slot open the very next morning at 7:30 a.m.; otherwise she wouldn't be able to do it for another week. It was all happening so fast, but somehow I trusted her and felt that I had put things off long enough. So I quickly said, "Let's do it tomorrow," and the next morning I had surgery.

The surgery is called tumor debulking. They cut me open from just under my bra to my bikini line and tried to cut out as much of the cancer as is visible to the eye. Then they hope the chemotherapy will wipe out the smaller, microscopic portions of the disease.

I was in the hospital for about a week. I had a tube going down my throat, which was just awful. The incision was very painful. I was so scared and sick. I wish I had a dollar for every time I vomited during that week. My husband slept in an uncomfortable chair, and it would give me comfort to wake up in the night and see him there. I began to feel human again once that throat tube was taken out and the vomiting subsided. On one of my worst days I looked up and there stood what looked like an angel to me. It was the chaplain of the hospital. It was dark in my room with only the light from the television on, but there she stood with her sweet, soft voice and her Bible in hand. She introduced herself and asked if I would like her to pray with me. I was raised as a Presbyterian but hadn't attended church on a regular basis since I was a child. Somehow, her offer of prayer made me feel that God had sent her to me. I welcomed her prayer, and she made me feel much calmer. She told me about a support group at Baylor for ovarian cancer patients. I took her card on which she had written the date and time of the meetings.

My son came to visit me every day in the hospital. I remember being quite confused about the presidential election. I kept asking him who had won. After all, it was about November 6th, and we should know by then. He kept telling me there was a glitch, and we didn't know yet. I would look at the television and still not quite understand why there was no named winner of the election yet. I now look back and think how the entire nation was confused at what was going on. It wasn't just me. I think my son inherited my love of the movies, and late one evening when he was getting up to leave, I said, "Hey, Mike, life is like a box of chocolates. You never know what you are going to get." He smiled big; he knew just what I meant. I took the line out of the movie *Forrest Gump*.

So after a week in the hospital, I finally got to go home. It never felt so good to get in my own bed and bathroom. Okay, now onto chemotherapy. I would start it right after Thanksgiving. I was still weak from surgery but started mentally preparing myself for the dreaded chemo and, gulp, losing my hair. I had seen versions of chemotherapy and the results of hair fallout in the movies, but I just could not imagine what it would be like. Would I look like Demi Moore in *GI Jane*? I was just trying to conjure up what it would be like to look at myself in the mirror with no hair. When I was diagnosed, my hair was long and highlighted blonde. I felt that my hair was my crowning glory, and that darned chemo was going to wipe out my glory.

My well-meaning sister offered to shave her head in a show of support. I rejected her offer, knowing that she would have fainted if I had taken her up on it. Several friends with good intentions said, "It won't be so bad." Yeah—right! I was unconvinced and knew they weren't the ones losing their hair. It was going to be horrific for me, and I knew it.

A couple of weeks after my first chemo treatment, my hair began to shed like a mangy dog. Once it started to fall out in big clusters, I went to my hair stylist and asked her to "buzz it off" near the scalp. During the buzzing, I was turned away from the mirror. When she finished and turned me around in the chair, I looked at my image in the mirror. Horrified at the sight of myself, I could barely bring myself to take a second look.

Now that I was bald, I decided my head had to be covered with something. I bought two wigs, which I quickly realized I would never bond with. Also, I purchased about a dozen hats, hoping that a few might be comfortable. I decided on a favorite hat, a black cotton knit one that became a fixture on my head. I let my granddaughter, Evan, play dress up with the others.

One day, Evan's curiosity got the best of her. She asked to look at my head underneath the hat. I showed her my shiny, hairless dome. She wasn't shocked at all. She looked carefully at my head and nonchalantly stated, "Don't worry, Nona, it will grow back." Somehow her honest remark was the most encouragement I had received from anyone. Out of the mouths of babes...

For solace, I turned to the women in the ovarian cancer support group, which I began attending just weeks after my surgery and before my first chemotherapy. Some wore wigs, others wore scarves and baseball caps. One spunky lady wore a cap that said "Wish You Were Hair." From observing them, I got an idea of what my options were.

I know some view support groups negatively. They think a bunch of people gather and cry the blues. I found quite the opposite. We have a great sense of camaraderie, share information, and have many laughs. I have found it to be extremely helpful. I have formed bonds with some of those women that are so strong. I feel that I have known them all my life. That support group became very important to me.

From November 2000 to April 2001, I did six treatments of chemotherapy called Taxol and carboplatin. I finished up chemo, and by August 2001, I had enough hair, albeit very short, to go public without a hat. I was feeling good.

I was sailing along, but then I began to worry about having a recurrence. That cloud seemed to loom over my head. Why couldn't I just not worry about it?

I read books, researched medical information, talked to survivors who lived 24/7 with the fear, and observed how the women in my support group were coping. My conclusions were that like many things in life, there is no "cookie-cutter" way to deal with the possibility of a recurrence. There is not a right way or a wrong way. We each have to deal with the fear of a recurrence in a way that helps us get through the day.

After a 9-month remission following initial chemotherapy, pain, blood test results, and a CT scan confirmed that the ovarian cancer was back. Shock was my first reaction, and then I was devastated. Although the possibility of a recurrence was ever present, I had lived those 9 months quite happily. I felt strong; hair was on my head; no way could it be back. I was scared and angry. I had done everything exactly as I was supposed to and yet still had a recurrence. Plus, I feared the unknown. What was going to happen next?

I started taking another chemotherapy drug called Doxil. After regular treatments, I stayed on Doxil for 3 years and 8 months. When it seemed not to be working as well, my doctor and I decided a vacation from chemo was in order. I went for 5 months before starting back on one of the original drugs, carboplatin. I've been on that since April 2006. So far, so good.

I continue to worry about another recurrence, especially on those days after I take the CA-125 blood test, when I anxiously wait for the results. For the most part, I take a deep breath, worry for a few days, and then get on with living.

My thoughts of "Will it come back, what will I do, just how sick will I get" took up a growing amount of my energy. So I answered those questions for myself. The answers being, yes, it is a possibility that it will come back. I am blessed with a superb doctor, nurses, and health facility. I will do the best I can with the tools I have. Chemotherapy is not a picnic in the park, but I will go through it and hope that the end will justify the means.

Sometimes I feel that there is a sleeping giant in my body just waiting to rear its ugly head. And if it does return, I will just do the best I can to continue fighting. I have been braver than I ever thought I was capable of being.

In the meantime I am just getting on with enjoying life. As the old song says, "Accentuate the positive, eliminate the negative, and don't mess with Mr. In Between." I try to stay away from people who are negative. I truly believe they are toxic to my system.

One of the most important purposes in my life is to love and be with my grandchildren. They are only 6 and 8, and when I teach them a life lesson, I feel such a sense of accomplishment. My soul feels such joy when I am around them, and I feel that my immune system benefits from that. I have started a Grandmother Journal full of my thoughts. Oh, how I wish I had something like that from my grandmother. I think to write a letter to someone you love is one of the best gifts you can give.

I've found helping others nourishes me in a special way. It makes me feel so worthy of being on this planet to be able to help a lady who also has ovarian cancer. I meet so many wonderful women through my support group and at the hospital where I am treated. We are all fighting in a war together, the war against cancer.

I count my blessings every day, as I know things can change in a minute and be gone with the wind. And on the days when I feel low, I just tell myself, "Tomorrow is another day."

Kay Knodel

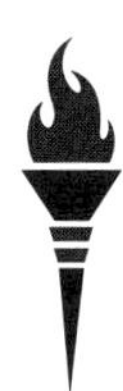

Twilight: The Soft Light Between Sunset and Darkness

I ONCE HEARD it said that you get shown the light in the strangest places if you look at it right. Well, after being diagnosed with stage III ovarian cancer in November 2000, a darkness enveloped my life like no other. I had previously experienced some stomach problems and had noticed a marble-sized lump visible near my navel. I was referred to a surgeon who promptly removed the lump and biopsied it. I received the numbing news that I had an offshoot of ovarian cancer. I began a regimen of six chemotherapy treatments and surgery followed by more chemo. I then experienced a 2-year remission from my enemy. After that seemingly brief hiatus, I had a recurrence that required more surgery and more chemotherapy. I was blessed to have another 2-year remission before the cancer recurred. Once again, more surgery and chemotherapy.

Just about the time I thought that the darkest of times might be over, I lost my best friend, my mother. This was in 2004. It was a painful time for me. But, I was fortunate to still have the most wonderful of husbands. Bruce and I had been married almost 51 years. We had two sons and a daughter and seven grandchildren. Bruce was experiencing a myriad of health issues of his own due to diabetes. However, he was my constant cheerleader during my illness. He was my small bit of light in an otherwise dark time. Nothing could have prepared me for the shock of his unexpected death during a hospital outpatient procedure. I took him to the hospital for the routine procedure. I just thought we would be going home afterward. It never dawned on me we wouldn't. I would, but Bruce wouldn't. How was I to summon the strength to continue? If God loves me, and I believe He does, why did this have to happen? We were just beginning 2006. It was off to an awful start.

While it has been difficult at times to keep up the continual fight against the cancer that preys on me, light has filtered through in various places. God had shown me how my children, grandchildren, doctors, friends, and of course, the ovarian cancer support group are there for me. Our loving leader, Jann, and the ladies in the group share a bond like no other. I consider them to be the sisters I never had. How ironic that I had been hesitant at first to attend a support meeting. I thought, "Who wants to be around other sick women?" If I look around, I can find the light. The blessings in my life and the weekly group meetings have proven to be just that. Blessings. Somehow I've earned the nickname "Strawberry Shortcake." It could be because of my height, or lack of it. I am called "Shortcake" and receive gifts of strawberry-themed cards, favors, and even bubble bath.

Another boost to my life are the twice-a-week line dancing classes I attend. We are all seniors, mostly women and three or four brave men. The movement, music, and rhythm assist in helping my mind focus away from the troubling thoughts. Other happy times are spent in the kitchen baking or cooking favorite dishes to share with family and friends. Thinking of others shifts my brain from thinking of myself.

I am fortunate in having two of my three children close by. My son lives in Dallas and my daughter in San Antonio. She makes frequent trips to Dallas to visit or to take me home with her for a few days. She's made it very comfortable for me. There are living quarters for me in back of her house. She keeps the fridge stocked with Blue Bell and sugar-free topping. I have everything I need there. And I have a standing invitation to come and make the move permanent. For now, I have elderly aunts here in Dallas, and I like knowing I can keep an eye on them and run errands when necessary. It's also nice to know I have a home when I am ready in San Antonio.

I would characterize my present status physically and emotionally as being in a twilight time. Twilight, that soft light between sunset and darkness. Today, at this moment I am considered stable. I have the highs and the lows. The joy and the depths of despair. For now, I am satisfied and thankful for being in between...in the twilight.

Elena Lowry

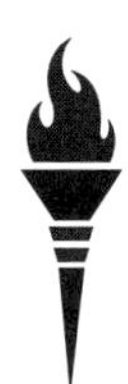

Into the Light

I BELIEVE in miracles. I believe in life after death. I believe that each of us owns a divine purpose in all our energy forms, and every circumstance is necessary down to the tiniest of details.

I did not always think exactly in this manner. This is a God-inspired philosophy that evolved over time. My worldly path there, like most, was not easy and is certainly ongoing. However, I will say I am a predominantly joyful person, full of hope. My family would lovingly (and proudly) tease me when I was a kid, saying, "Lora always sticks up for the underdog!" My beautiful sister adds, " …perpetually looking at the world with rose-colored glasses." They're right. This is how I choose to live. How I choose to see humanity. How I cherish myself and the ones I love.

Please don't misunderstand; it is impossible to ignore all the sorrow and suffering of this world. It's just that I know we have unimaginable power as human beings to make our hearts and this world a better place. Despite crime, inequality, hunger, war, poverty, evil, hate, deception, abuse…despite cancer.

I believe in second chances. I believe there is always light at the end of even the darkest of tunnels. I believe that I can do anything through Christ who lives in my heart, making me pure and beautiful and smart and the woman that I am.

When I was 26 years old, I began suffering from symptoms of ovarian cancer. Three years later I was wheeled into surgery to remove what were thought to be benign cysts. I came out of that hospital with a whole new life. Gone was the false sense of security of good health. Gone was the dream of ever having children of my own. Gone was a smooth belly without scarring and adhesions. I had cancer. That was a lot to understand.

So began my journey toward recovery. The pig-headed Lora has a huge sense of independence and a wild streak that feeds an incredibly insatiable desire for adventure. No fear. Huge confidence. No regrets. Gone was the pig-headed Lora. I was scared. I was sad. I felt alone.

I believe God gives you what you need at every turn. I believe that when we love one another and expect the very best, people are innately good. I believe none of us are perfect, but we have a responsibility to do the right thing.

Friends, I have lied, cheated, stolen, cussed, smoked, drank. I have prayed, loved, supported, dreamed, given, thanked. Until cancer, I had always known who I am, whether acting out or acting right. After that diagnosis, I froze in my grief and despair and fear. I was lost, confused, wedged. And, it was odd that I found myself in the basement of a hospital, attending an ovarian cancer support group, but those women changed my life in so many wonderful ways.

I learned how to reinvent myself, put others before me, express my pain, cry and laugh again. I learned how to honor my body, delight in my gifts, cherish and forgive. I learned how to dream again, have hope, give back, accept my loss and soar. I learned that I am special if I set myself apart and that cancer makes me stronger, not weaker. I learned that I am brave, unique, blessed and beautiful despite my scars. I learned it is okay to be sad and angry but better to do something about it for good. I learned every day is a gift, and I have an incredible family and a loving and kind husband.

I believe that there is always someone who has a worse set of circumstances than my own. I believe that what we give, God gives us back tenfold. I believe that when the fog of fear is lifted, we have an amazing glimpse at paradise.

My ovarian cancer support group sisters mean more to me than they would ever imagine. They have taught me so much and encourage me in everything I undertake. I carry each of them in my heart and am so grateful to have known every one of these darling warriors. They are my inspiration, my hope, my reason, and a gift far beyond measure. I love them. I thank them. I rejoice in their beauty. They make me not afraid.

I believe that when I die, I will have eternal life. I believe that in heaven, God will let me help paint the sunsets. I believe that in spirit form I will have

a greater ability to love and guide and protect those who are most important
to me.

Lora Swanson Williams

— 89 —

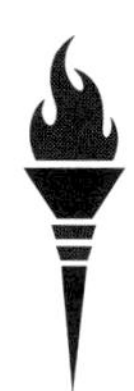

The "Son"Shine Connection

Blessed be the God and Father of our Lord Jesus Christ, the Father of mercies and God of all comfort; who comforts us in all our affliction so that we may be able to comfort those who are in any affliction with the comfort with which we ourselves are comforted by God" (2 Corinthians 1:3–4).

WHEN CRISIS COMES and emotions crumble, questions multiply. We may ask: How can I cope? What next? God, where are you? Is there light at the end of this tunnel? The past 2½ years I have been acquainted with women who ask similar questions.

When I know someone else survived an experience, and I find myself in a similar situation, I feel that I can survive, too. This is the reason I joined the Cvetko support group at Baylor in Dallas, Texas. It is my hope that sharing my experience with ovarian cancer will help you with your personal journey with this disease.

I was caregiver for my mother for some years before a crippling stroke left her totally dependent on others for her care. My mother needed constant care for a year before the Lord took her home. My body was reeling from incredible stress, depression, and fatigue after Mom died. In August 2004, 11 months after my mother's death, I was diagnosed with stage IIIC ovarian cancer. I had visited my family doctor in June, July, and August 2004 with complaints of abdominal pain, swelling, indigestion, nausea, extreme fatigue, and the inability to empty my bladder. My doctor ran a urine test and said it was negative for any type of infection. He went on to tell me it was probably my age (60 years old) and/or the heat of the Texas summer getting to me. I thanked him and left his office knowing full well it was not my imagination. The doctor caught up with me before I left his office and suggested that I have a vaginal sonogram. I told him I had an appointment with my gynecologist in Dallas the next day, and I would ask her to do the test. (After all, I was thinking, you have had 3 months to do something.)

That evening I prayed for God's help. Unable to sleep I got out of bed and looked for my *Mayo Clinic Health Book*. For some reason I started looking at female cancers. There it was: "ovarian cancer." My immediate response was "Oh my God! Do I have ovarian cancer?"

The next day, as I drove to Dallas to see my gynecologist, all I could think of was the possibility of cancer. As I told my doctor of my symptoms (not mentioning what I had read in the *Mayo Clinic Health Book* the night before), I saw the concerned look on her face. I could tell I was in trouble. Even before the doctor examined me, based on my symptoms, she said she was afraid it could be ovarian cancer. The pelvic exam did not indicate any unusual findings. Off to x-ray I went for the vaginal sonogram. When the x-ray technician was finished, she sent me back to my doctor's office. When Dr. Roe entered into her personal office, where I was, she chose to sit beside me and not at her desk. She took my hand and told me it was ovarian cancer. She went on to say it appeared to be late stage. I noticed tears collecting in her eyes. Thank you, God, for doctors who see me not only as a patient but as a person. She told me that she knew a gynecologic oncologist that she would like to recommend for me to see. I asked her to make the appointment with this Dr. Fine and left her office, assuring her I was able to drive myself home. As I drove home, 60 miles east of Dallas, I prayed for wisdom to tell my husband, Jim, and our daughter, Stephanie, about my serious disease.

How can I cope? Prayer for me is very important. I immediately asked my family, friends, and my church family to pray for me and my family. I had surgery within 7 days of my diagnosis. I had confidence in Dr. Fine as my surgeon. After all, I had asked God for the best doctor and nurses to surround me. Family and friends took turns taking care of me after surgery. A couple of days after surgery, Dr. Fine came into my hospital room to explain to me what to expect in the upcoming months of treatment. He told me I would start chemo treatments within 3 weeks with Taxol and carboplatin, the standard treatment for ovarian cancer. Then Dr. Fine went on to tell me that he would like for me to go to M. D. Anderson for a protocol trial including high-dose chemo/ autologous bone marrow transplant. To qualify for this protocol I would have to have a second-look surgery after I finished the chemo. He also said he would like for me to talk to one of his patients who had finished the trial at M. D. Anderson. He said she could help me with valuable information. Debby, the patient Dr. Fine told me about, called after I was home from surgery. Her voice was so compassionate, and her story of experience was reassuring. She told me of her remission since her treatment at M. D. Anderson. She shared what I could expect there and helped with valuable information. Debby also encouraged me to attend the ovarian cancer support group at Baylor.

I had a second-look surgery on February 14, 2005. All the biopsies showed no cancer. Our insurance said the M. D. Anderson trial was experimental and investigational and denied me coverage. My husband's company stepped in and made my trip to M. D. Anderson possible in July 2005. As I prepared for my Houston trip, I was told I would need caregivers for 9 weeks. My first thought was: Where am I going to get all this help? My daughter, in Indiana, has two small children to care for. My husband, chief pilot for his company, could not be away from his job for that long. The news traveled fast to family and friends for my needs for the M. D. Anderson trip. Calls came pouring in. Within a very short time my needs were met and a complete schedule of care-givers that included family and friends was in place. My husband filled in the gaps as needed. He came nearly every week to shuttle caregivers and encourage me along the way. Many others, too many to name, were so supportive with food, cards, and e-mails. The bond I share with all these people who blessed me with their skills of caregiving is amazing. After 9 weeks at M. D. Anderson, I went home September 2, 2005. I was very weak but very hopeful that this treatment would allow me a long remission or, even better, a cure.

What next? In February 2006, my CA-125 was 12.7. This was great. Then a month went by, and it was up to 17.2. Another month went by, and it was 26.4. When the CA-125 reached 31.9 in June 2006, Dr. Fine said he believed I was in recurrence. My CT scans showed nothing for the past few months. Dr. Fine said, "Betty, we need to start treatment." I said, "Hold on.

I need more than the CA-125 rising to convince me that 'it' is back." A PET scan was ordered, and it showed a hot spot in my lower right abdomen, where the appendix used to be. The appendix was cancerous and removed with the initial surgery. Dr. Fine thought this was the beginning of my recurrence. I let him know I was ready to start treatments.

I delayed treatments for a month. I had promised my two small grand-children, earlier in the year, that they could come and stay with Nana and Papa for a month for their summer vacation. On August 26, 2006, I started chemo treatments. Dr. Fine's choice for treatment was carboplatin. Because my platelets went down to 18, he recommended a different chemotherapy. By September, after trying two treatments of Doxil, my CA-125 had risen to 108. Because of the rapid increase of my CA-125, the Doxil treatment was discontinued. My CT scan was still negative in November. This was very troubling because I wanted to see what I was fighting. In November, we started treatments of cisplatin/Gemzar, and my CA-125 was up to 147. By the time I had my second treatment using cisplatin/Gemzar, my platelets were down to 16.

Another CT scan was done on January 3, 2007. Finally, the cancer showed itself. Dr. Fine called me late that night to tell me that my CT scan was not good. He had conferred with another surgeon. The cancer was covering the left side of my intestines and colon. It was inoperable. Dr. Fine said he would like me to see a Dr. Bevers in Houston, as he felt he had done all he could for me. Dr. Bevers is connected with M. D. Anderson, and Dr. Fine said he would know of various trials available there, and he also specialized in unusual cases such as mine. My husband and I stayed up most of that night. We held each other, crying and praying.

God, where are you? That Sunday Jim and I went to our evening Bible study group and shared the latest news with them. The women and men in this group have been our faithful prayer warriors ever since my diagnosis. That night they all placed their emotions before God, asking for a miracle for me. After our prayers, I felt the peace that can only come from God. The next morning I woke up and had the strangest thing happen. I felt as if someone had "slapped" me on the forehead. Just then my thought was to go and see Dr. Bevers in Houston for a second opinion. A couple of hours passed. My daughter called and said she had talked to Dr. Fine. He told her he really wanted me to go to see this doctor in Houston. Stephanie went on to say, "Mom, you need to get another opinion."

The next day I called Becky, one of my dear friends in my support group, and I shared the news of the CT scan with her. As always she reassured me with scriptures of God's promises to me. Becky is always there with hope when I need it. She is amazing. You see, she has her own battle with ovarian cancer, but she always finds time to lift me as well as others in the group up when we need it most. She is one of those helpers I prayed for God to send.

Becky sent out an e-mail to the support group, asking for prayer for me. The next morning was a cold, damp, overcast day. I made a cup of coffee and went out to my back patio to talk to God. I reached up to the heavens, my hands outstretched, and cried, "God, please help me! Send me some sunshine today to let me know you are here with me!" I knew the warmth of the sun would assure me He was near. I finished my cup of coffee and prayers and went inside. Just then the phone rang. It was Becky. She called to make sure that I was okay. After we finished our talk, my phone rang again. This was Dody, also from the support group. Dody is a 17-year survivor of ovarian cancer! She is a beacon of hope for all of us. As we talked, she also encouraged me to go and see the doctor in Houston for another opinion. Dody was sharing scripture with me when all of sudden I realized that God had just sent me the "sunshine" I had asked Him for. Becky and Dody were His gift of sunshine for me that day. I was still sitting in the rocking chair in my bedroom when another amazing thing happened. This brilliant sunshine broke out of the clouds, filling my bedroom with its luminous light. I choked back my tears. God is once again letting me know He is so very near to me today.

Thank you, God, for the "Son"shine (Jesus) that is in my life every day.

My visit with Dr. Bevers in Houston went well. He said he believed the stem cell transplant with all the chemo had damaged my bone marrow. He did have some suggestions for Dr. Fine in reference to my treatments. I also had a call from Dr. Fine's office, letting me know that my CA-125 had dropped from 149 to 63. It was amazing that the little chemo we were able to get into me was indeed working. Jim and I left from Houston with renewed hope for my treatments.

I had two more cisplatin and Gemzar treatments, which were lowered by 20%, per Dr. Bevers' instruction. We really hoped this would not cause my platelets to "crash." However, my platelets went down to 16. I had to have a platelet transfusion. Three weeks passed with no chemo because my platelets were still down. In the meantime, my daughter and grandchildren came from Indiana for a visit I really needed. Dr. Fine and I were discussing my chemo schedule or the lack of one when I told him that my family was the best medicine for me at this time. I know he is really concerned for me not being on a schedule and I am too, but I know it will all work out.

Is there light at the end of this tunnel? Dr. Fine just called. I felt immediately it was bad news about my recent CA-125. No, he is happy! Really happy! "Betty, I am looking at your CA-125 and it is 23!" I asked him, "Are you sure, Dr. Fine? Are you sure you are looking at my lab work?" "Yes," he concurred. I started crying. I have not allowed myself to cry in front of Dr. Fine before now. I explained to Dr. Fine these are tears of joy!! There was a pause. Dr. Fine said, "Well, I will go now before you have me crying." Is he not precious?

As you face the hills and valleys set before you, it is my hope that this prayer will provide you with some "Son"shine along the way. "God, you know my feelings are going haywire; they scream and shout that this situation is terrible and there is no hope. God, I hope in you. I can't see what You are doing, but I trust that You are working this situation together for good. Thank you that you have promised to use it to make me more like Christ. This is what I want…. It just doesn't feel good today. Give me the strength to focus my eyes on You and not on what I can see. Amen."

Betty Skinner

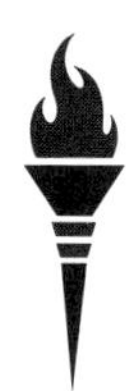

"On a Bumpy Road with Ovarian Cancer"
with Jesus Driving and Me, Dody Stovall, Riding Shotgun

THIS JOURNEY of mine began in January 1990, when I went into surgery for a routine hysterectomy and came out with a diagnosis of ovarian cancer, stage IIIA. I was put in the hands of a wise and wonderful gynecologic oncologist, and we have walked this road together for 17 years, while fighting for my life.

Back in the early days before Taxol and all the wonderful nausea meds, I was given suppositories before and after chemo. I would go home and sleep for 18 to 20 hours to keep my body quiet and not be so nauseated. Two months after surgery, after I had done two rounds of chemo, I asked Dr. Stringer if I could go skiing, and he looked at me, grinned, and said, "You can't stop living, Dody, but promise me that you will stay on the bunny slope and don't fall on your butt" (in my family we say "bokey"). I took four more rounds of chemo, and then I was in a 6-year remission period and dancing with NED (no evidence of disease).

At this point, my wonderful supportive family decided to give me a "No Mo Chemo" party and rented a big house down in the Hill Country. The in-laws and out-laws came to celebrate with costumes, songs, poems, and even a skit with "Dr. Stringer," scrubs and all, chasing the so-called "me" with a huge syringe and needle that was a foot long. It was wonderful to feel good again.

Then, during a routine exam, a tumor was found. Once again, I had surgery plus six more months of chemo. This time I got to take Taxol. My hair began falling out, and I decided the best thing to do was to shave it. I asked my husband, Joe, to help me, and he was appalled. I put a chair on the deck and draped a towel around me, and he started cutting until nary a hair was left. Then he took a step backward, looked at me, and said, "Now, I don't want you cavorting with the Germans anymore!" I laughed until I was weak as pond water. It wasn't long before the hair was coming back in curly, and once again I was feeling good and started on another long remission of 5 years.

Two years later I was "on the road again" with another recurrence, but this time surgery wasn't an option, and we started playing the chemo game. Some working and some not. Now the goal is to keep me stable, and that's fine with me. Hope and stable are two beautiful words.

While I was taking my very first chemo, Dr. Stringer said he had plans for me to start working with his patients to get to know them and become their friend since there was little or no support for ovarian cancer patients. This opened up a new ministry for me and changed my life forever. I saw everything clearly through different eyes as these girls were transparent, and I could see into their hearts and feel their fear. As I visited in their hospital rooms, seeds were sown spiritually and physically, and our bonds grew strong. Soon I was having luncheons for them and weekend retreats in my home.

Another turn in my road came when the Baylor ovarian cancer support group was formed about a year after my original diagnosis, and that was a Godsend. At long last the girls had a place of their own to come and pour out their hearts. The group has changed many times through the years, and each girl has been unique and a real blessing. I've kept picture albums of the girls, and it's a nostalgic moment to sit and look at each face and "remember."

In spite of all the needles, drips, nausea, lack of energy, loss of hair and dignity, and the dread of the difficulty of dying, God always makes something good come from something bad, so the blessings far outweigh the problems. We're here as a group to comfort and encourage one another, and I think we do a beautiful job of that. Each girl is so easy to love, so TLC comes naturally. We have to remember on this journey where we came from and what we've learned so we can pass it on to the newbies, and they in turn can pass it on to others.

Before I ever started this journey, my ticket was already bought by God's amazing grace through His Son, so I'm really home free. Come on…climb aboard with me, and let's travel this road together, and believe it or not, we're going to have some fun along the way no matter how many bumps are in the road.

Dody Stovall

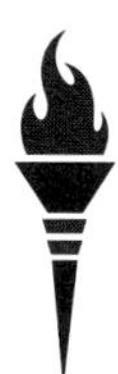

Sailing, Sailing

I STARTED my ovarian cancer journey on May 14, 2004. There had been no cancer in my family, so my annual gynecological appointment was quite a shock. I think I was in shock for several months. We had a vacation planned, leaving 3 days later. I opted not to tell Joe, my husband, the news until we got back. I worry about his working too hard, so I wanted us to enjoy the trip. I will always be glad it worked out. He had a great time and so did I on our cruise out of Galveston.

My first operation was on June 2, 2004. The cancer was stage IIIC and quite extensive. I understand now how important it is to have a gynecologic oncologist take charge! I had never heard of debulking but realized after much reading that it is a big factor. One ovary was against the colon, so a large section had to be removed and reconnected. Six days later, the connection leaked, and a colostomy was performed. That extended my shock. A reversal was discussed for the following summer, which gave me some hope. Hope is a big, strong word and feeling in this journey.

I went to support groups near my home but found a wonderful group at the Cvetko Center at Baylor Hospital. I cannot find the words to describe my experience, but the group has done so much for me. I also joined an ostomy group that helped me settle down in that aspect. I got a book on traveling with a colostomy. In February, my doctor let me have a month off chemotherapy to go on our annual sailing trip. I was on Taxol for maintenance, and I did just fine. The colostomy nurse was so caring and helped me a great deal. Putting the bag on and keeping the skin clear was a full-time job. That seemed an unreal part of my life.

I had the colostomy reversed that summer. During the last few months, I had developed a hernia at the site, the first of many hernias. Although the scan was clear, the doctor said he had found numerous small cancers during surgery. I was so disheartened to learn that the scan had been clear, but I needed to start back on chemotherapy. I finished that in October, and in January we went sailing again. There were two couples, and we were sailing in the British Virgin Islands. We were relaxed and had a good time. Joe and I make good crewmen. It was a wonderful experience. Returning, we shocked our family. Joe had grown a full beard, and my very short hair surprised them. We had been gone a month. I wish I had a picture of their expressions.

I had been working out with a trainer before cancer and kept it up. She took it easy with me. I felt much better then than I do now. I damaged some tendons and ligaments in my foot. I did not want to do surgery. I quit exercising, and that was a big mistake. I read many books on hope, spirituality, and the mind-body connection. I feel a good outlook is essential.

I was uplifted by cards and flowers from old friends and new. I was in the hospital for 3 weeks and enjoyed all the flowers. Now I have quite a collection of baskets. I appreciate life, friends, and family so much more now. A good first read is Lance Armstrong's *It's Not About the Bike.*

My third summer I had a large hernia where I had gone through emergency surgery 20 years ago. During the surgery for the hernia, my doctor put in a port for IP chemo, interperitoneal infusion. On my third treatment, we found there were too many adhesions, so it was back to the veins. Soon I was feeling awful, not eating and in pain. A scan showed a colon blockage and stones in my gallbladder. Of course, a hernia, too. I went into the hospital for exploratory surgery. I had lost a lot of weight, so I had to build my body back up. I had the surgery for the blockage the day before Halloween. The IP tubing had been wrapped around my colon.

My chemotherapy had been interrupted, so I was off schedule. I opted not to go on our annual January sailing trip. It was the first one we had missed in 10 years. It was a good thing we stayed home. On January 14, 2007, I had to have emergency gallbladder surgery. The surgery started at 6:00 in the evening. It was supposed to be 2 hours but went for 4½ hours.

I have to thank my husband, Joe, for his help, cheerfulness, and good humor. I cannot imagine going through this without him. I enjoy being spoiled.

I rest, play Sodoku, and read. I don't cook. Joe does cook, and he was glad when I started going back to the grocery store and cleaning the kitchen. He appreciates how much there is to do in a home. My children have been here for me. My sailing buddies have taught me how to be a hugger. My reticent son even hugs me now. Good things do come out of bad. My daughter plays Sodoku and likes to read, so she is good company. My children, their spouses, and my grandchildren have all done their share. I enjoy their company.

I didn't dwell on my fatigue. It's always there, some days more than others. I like the saying, "the new normal." That is so true. I am on a single chemo agent now, Gemzar. I realized as I was writing my story how much I have been able to do in spite of ovarian cancer! I have a wonderful family and friends. My good humor is a gift. On most days, I am sailing!

Jill Park

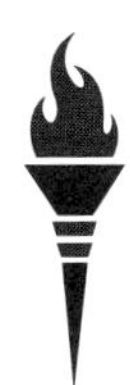

Normal: Just a Setting on My Washer

OR MONTHS after I was diagnosed with stage IIIC ovarian cancer in December 1997, I counted the days until I healed from my surgery, made it through each round of chemotherapy, drank my last batch of contrast fluid, and made it through the anxiety of another checkup.... All I could think of was when I get finished with all these treatments, my life will get back to normal. As I neared the end of my chemo and first line of treatment, I began to panic. How was I going to do this on my own? Man, I needed those drugs to keep the cancer away. At some point it dawned on me that here I was asking to stay on chemo when I had been counting the days until it ended, because then I could get back to normal. Over the period of a few days I began to realize that the normal I knew before cancer was gone forever. My tears flowed for days on end as I grieved the loss of an innocent, carefree way of life that I never really appreciated. I somehow understood that my diagnosis would become a part of the fabric of my life.

Nine years, 3 months, and 21 days have passed since my diagnosis. I consider myself well, but not cured. I am not sure one is ever cured of ovarian cancer until you die of something else. That horrible nickname of "the silent killer" haunts me to this day. I like that we now refer to it as the disease "that whispers."

My affair with ovarian cancer came as a complete surprise. After what I thought was a routine hysterectomy to remove a large fibroid tumor, an unknown doctor appeared in recovery to tell me I had ovarian cancer and was going to have 6 months of chemo and lose all of my hair. My husband and ob-gyn saw me briefly and left. Somehow, I survived that first night and the following weeks.

The unknown doctor in recovery turned out to be a gynecologic oncologist from Texas Oncology, Dr. Alan Gordon. My longtime ob-gyn had called him to do my surgery when he saw it looked like ovarian cancer. For this I will be eternally grateful because several years later I read that if an ovarian cancer patient has her surgery done by a gynecologic oncologist, her chances of survival are eight times greater. In those days I grasped at any bit of positive information.

At our meeting with Dr. Gordon to discuss chemo, my husband Ray and I were shocked to hear the survival rates using what he called the "gold standard," Taxol and carboplatin. We pressed him for other alternatives. He finally offered us a chance to use three chemo drugs instead of two, but they had to be alternated because using all three at once would kill me. The routine was to be eight rounds of chemo using Taxol/carboplatin alternated with Taxol/topotecan. Topotecan was still in the trial stages and not yet FDA approved. Something about attacking the cancer cells three different ways appealed to us. We both felt instantly comfortable with this choice. A peace came to us about these drugs. We never once looked back.

I was labeled Topotecan 6. With the use of this drug, I got a wonderful research nurse, Julie Boston, who would walk with me, and close monitoring by Dr. Gordon because the research project required it. For me this was all a wonderful blessing since I am one who needs tons of information.

Ray decided I would never be left alone during chemo treatments. He came with me and stayed the entire time, sometimes 10 hours. He also felt each of our five children should be with me through at least one session so they would understand what I was going through. I loved having each of them with me. A bonding took place during these sessions, and I soon understood that it was not just me who had ovarian cancer. Our whole family had it, too, and we were all in this fight together. For the first time in my life, I felt so valued and loved by these kids and their dad. It was awesome. I began to understand that there were blessings that came with a life-threatening diagnosis. We pulled together like we had never done before. Each of us had to redefine "what matters most" in our lives.

In my crisis over wanting my old normal back, Dr. Gordon told me I could not stay on chemo forever. Again, I pushed him for other alternatives. Surely there was something else I could do to keep this disease at bay. Again, Dr. Gordon offered me a chance at a drug trial for a monoclonal antibody called OvaRex. It was a double-blind study. I might get the drug and I might not, but I didn't care. I wanted to do the drug trial, and I did. Once again I got fantastic follow-up, CAT scans, and checkups that continued for 5 years. About the time the OvaRex follow-up was ending, Dr. Gordon told me he was moving to Phoenix to head a research program there. Even being 5 years out, I felt my main supporter was being removed. Fortunately, Dr. Allen Stringer stepped in to keep me going, and he weaned me off my endless checkups.

I was young, only 54 years old, and had never been ill....

I knew from Dr. Gordon that my chances of a recurrence were over 40%, but I decided that I was going to be in that 60% that did not have a recurrence. Any time there was something negative, I found a way to turn it into a positive. If the OvaRex was given to 50%, then I was one who got it.

I decided if I had one day, one month, or one year to live, I would not spend one minute of it crying. I was going to enjoy every minute of each day.

I painted a rock with "What matters most?" on it and put it on my kitchen counter as a reminder to make that decision each day.

Ray and I made a "blessing bracelet" for me to wear every day so when I was afraid I would have an instant reminder of the blessings I had that cancer could not change. It had a cross to remind me of my faith, a heart to remind me of my love for God and my family and friends and their love for me, an angel to remind me I was never alone, and a dove to remind me of the peace I would have if I remembered the other three. After 5 years, we added an anchor as a symbol of hope for long-term survival. Last year we added a butterfly after I completed a personal growth program called The Barnabas Journey to symbolize the new way I was going to do life.

I decided that fear was a bigger killer than cancer; I had no room for it.

I prayed and meditated often.

I wrote daily in a journal and still do.

I sat in what I call the sun's healing rays.

I read and reread a book called *Everyday Strength: A Cancer Patient's Guide to Spiritual Survival* by Randy Becton.

I stopped drinking tap water.

I told my family and friends that I loved them. I hugged them often.

I went to the Baylor ovarian cancer support group and loved fellow fighters.

I became an advocate for my own health. I asked questions and more questions and got copies of my CAT scan reports and blood tests.

I argued with Ray for weeks about how we should do life. I wanted to slow down and run and play because I might not have time to do it in the future. But he couldn't do that. He felt that if we changed the way we did things, it would be like telling God we did not believe I was going to survive. We eventually had to do life differently from each other. He plodded along doing the usual routine. I ran off and played with my daughter and grandkids.

I found a wonderful psychologist to help me learn new ways to think.

I listened when Dr. Gordon got angry because I wanted to know statistics. He told me, "Statistics are just statistics." How could he compare me to a group that contains an 80-year-old woman, a 65-year-old woman who had heart disease for 20 years, a 70-year-old woman who never had regular checkups, or a 20-year-old college student? For statistics to be accurate, we would all have to be the same age and weight and have the same medical history and type of ovarian cancer. From that day forward, I forgot about statistics.

Today, March 27, 2007, I am alive, well, 63+ years old, working, and still longing for the normal that slipped away with that diagnosis of ovarian cancer. I have had to accept that I am happier when I believe that normal is really just a setting on my washing machine.

Peggy Hill

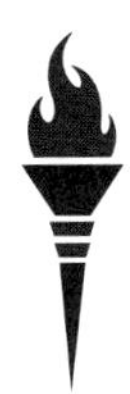

One Miracle
After Another

2006…what a year. I just entered my 40s and would describe myself as extremely fit and feeling great. In fact, I worked out several times a week and bragged to my husband and friends that I felt better than I ever did in my 30s.

I'm happily married with a 6-year-old kindergarten boy and still trying to figure out what I want to be when I grow up. You know, my passion. It's always stressed me out because deep in my heart I know that God put me on this earth to do something special. What that is, I still don't know, but I hope to discover it immediately.

I grew up in a small town in Oklahoma, with two brothers who were much older than I. We weren't extremely close because of our age differences, but that changed when my mother died suddenly in September 1997. It was so shocking and rocked my world. Our family got much tighter after that. We all learned that life is short and that you have to live each day to its fullest. I was 32, not married, and had just started a great new job after completing my MBA. I had to pick up the pieces and move on after the tragedy. Family support was vital in getting through it all.

So many things began happening after that event. I became engaged to Chris in 1998; got married in 1999; bought our first home; had a baby, Jacob, in 2000; lost my grandfather in 2001. You get the picture. While these events were happening, I was also experiencing my greatest career success ever. I traveled all over the world, had a ton of fun, and received a lot of praise from peers and company leaders.

Then, September 11th happened, and the company I worked for was negatively impacted. I didn't feel those impacts directly, but the mood around the organization and the constant layoffs took a toll on everyone. I started feeling that there was more to life and that I was missing out on being a mother to my son. So, at the end of 2002, I decided to be a stay-at-home mom. I have always been a conservative person, and this was the biggest risk I had ever taken, giving up a six-figure salary and not knowing my next step. But, I am glad I did, knowing what I know now.

It was wonderful to relive being 2, 3, 4, and 5 again. I can tell you that nothing makes me feel better than having one-on-one time with Jacob. I love him more than anything and have truly enjoyed teaching him skills and important life lessons. My prayer to God is that I can see my son grow up and become a man. I want to be influential in molding him to be an inspired human, with a strong faith in God, desire to be successful, and a genuinely empathetic person. The greatest gift for me would be to see Jacob get married and for me to become a grandmother, since my mother did not have that opportunity with me.

This leads me to 2006. My husband and I enjoy a wonderful life; we've been very lucky so far, although he just lost his mother after a long illness. We finally bit the bullet and purchased our second home. This one had good bones but needed a ton of work. It had the square footage, location, style, and potential we had been looking for so long. We felt it was the right one. Not so sure anymore.

Since we bought this house, we've had a small fire; nothing was really damaged, and we weren't living there at the time. We battled bad contractors before moving in. And then, only a week and a half after we moved in, we got the worst news of all.

I had been stressed with the move and dealing with the horrible contractors and wasn't sleeping or eating right. I didn't feel right and was having stomach issues. My family actually has a history with digestive problems. I never go to the doctor and have actually never had much of a reason because I'm rarely sick. The only doctor I even have is a gynecologist.

My stomach started to feel and look bloated. After much pleading from my dad and husband, I called my gynecologist. He told me to come in for a sonogram, since I was due for one anyway, and that he would probably send me to a gastroenterologist.

My appointment was September 8, 2006. I will never forget that day as long as I live. After the sonogram, I met my doctor in his office, and he proceeded to tell me I had ovarian cancer. What? I thought I had constipation. Cancer never crossed my mind in a million years. I knew he had to be wrong. He went on to share with me that one of my ovaries was the size of a grapefruit when it should be the size of an almond. Then he proceeded to tell me I needed to see an oncologist who would want to surgically remove everything, including all my female organs.

Wow! Never expected this. How could this be? I just saw this doctor in March, and I was told I was in excellent health. He gave me an A+. How could it change so dramatically in 6 months?

Apparently, that's the deal with ovarian cancer. It sneaks up on women with little to no recognizable symptoms. And, the gynecological medical community doesn't do any regular screening for it. Pap smears don't catch it, and I don't know of any doctors who run a CA-125 blood test annually. No wonder so many women die once diagnosed.

Once I got the news, panic and fear set in. I had to find a gynecologic oncologist, which was much tougher than expected. There aren't many around, but that was the type of doctor I wanted and needed. Most doctors in Dallas had at least a 2- to 3-week wait before I could get in for a consultation. But, God was watching out for me and provided my first miracle.

My sister-in-law in Houston is a nurse, and she happened to call on Friday, just 2 days after my diagnosis. She was in a state of shock as well. For some reason she had an administrative meeting the next day, Saturday, with the entire top management of the clinic she works for. She started talking to one of the VPs and mentioned she was distraught because of my situation. As fate would have it, this woman told her she was married to a gynecologic oncologist at M. D. Anderson and offered to have him call me over the weekend. He called me right away and invited me to come to his office that Tuesday for an examination and consultation. Wow! I couldn't believe it. How lucky to get into one of the most renowned cancer institutions and get one of the busiest surgeons in the department.

I made the appointment Monday, and my husband and I took off for Houston. Tuesday was an incredibly long day. We started at 7:30 a.m. and didn't leave the facility until 11:30 p.m. We first met Dr. Pedro Ramirez because he just came in to introduce himself. He was a very kind and, I must say, handsome young doctor. My sister-in-law and husband agreed. What a nice surprise.

The day was filled with lots of activity. First, the examination, follow-up consultation, EKG, blood test, and finally a lengthy 3-hour process for a CAT scan. I was exhausted and ready to get out of there.

I was scheduled to go back the next morning for another exam but opted not to go. I had another doctor to meet with in Dallas at 11:00 a.m. So, we caught an early flight back and then went to meet with another oncologist referred by my gynecologist. He was also very nice and very experienced.

Once my CAT scan results came back, I was given even more bad news. The cancer had spread extensively, and it was stage IV. The main concern was that it had potentially entered my liver, and they wouldn't know until they opened me up. I was told it would be a lengthy surgery. The surgeon at M. D. Anderson was very aggressive. He told me that once they opened me up, if they did not feel they could get the tumors down to <1 cm, they wouldn't move forward, and I would start chemotherapy. The Dallas doctor felt he could get 90% of the tumor. It was great to have another doctor to compare thoughts and tactics with. Ultimately, I decided to choose the M. D. Anderson route.

Surgery was scheduled for September 18th, the day before my son's birthday. I wanted to start my new life on his birthday. My whole family came to the hospital to wait. I was in surgery for 6 to 7 hours, but the outcome was the best we could hope for.

Dr. Ramirez believed he got everything. The cancer had not penetrated my liver, and I avoided bowel reconstruction surgery. Miracle number two. Hurray! I had a new lease on life.

I spent 21 days at M. D. Anderson; then upon my release I developed an awful infection which sent me back into the hospital on two different occasions. After about 6 weeks, I got stronger and was able to begin chemo-therapy.

My chemotherapy treatments were done in Dallas with Dr. Fine. He is also a wonderful doctor. I did extremely well through my six rounds, avoiding any illness, and stayed on track throughout the process.

February 8, 2007, was my last treatment, and on February 26, 2007, I got the most wonderful news ever. I am now cancer free! Miracle number three.

I feel that I owe my life to Dr. Ramirez, Dr. Fine, and Dr. Ted Fogwell, who also helped me with decision-making and desperate health crises during the recovery from surgery. This experience has strengthened my faith in God because I found out he really does perform miracles.

My cancer journey will continue as I fight to continue remission. I will do everything possible to make sure the cancer monster, as my son and I have deemed it, does not come back ever again. Maybe through this experience I will finally find my passion. I believe that may be God's plan.

I pray for all others who are also participating in this journey. They say what doesn't kill you makes you stronger. All cancer survivors truly know what that means.

Cindy Bartkoski

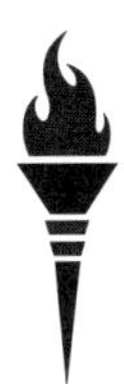

Counting My Blessings

I WAS 42 years old, and I had no idea I had cancer. I attended a baby shower on October 17, 2005, and when I returned home, I began to have pain in my abdomen. I was unable to sleep all night and contacted the physician on call on Sunday, October 18, 2005. After taking antibiotics and still not feeling any better on Monday, I called my physician. He recommended I go see him that morning. By that Monday morning my abdomen had started swelling.

My regular doctor recommended I see my gynecologist. After doing so, it was recommended I have a sonogram and CT scan. Before I received the results of the tests, I went to lunch with my mom and sister. As I was eating lunch, I received a phone call from my boss's wife asking how I was doing. She was vice president of a physicians' group for a local hospital system. She recommended I see an oncologist and told me she would make sure I could get in to see an oncology specialist. I called and was able to get an appointment.

I believe God was working in my life during this time. I initially had an appointment with my regular gynecologist, who had recommended surgery. Prior to the phone call from my boss's wife, I had planned to have a regular physician perform my surgery and had cancelled an appointment with the specialist. After my boss's wife called, I called the specialist back and my appointment had been given to another patient. The nurse said if I could come in at 7:30 a.m. the next morning (Friday, October 22, 2005), the oncologist would see me.

I believe God stepped in at this point to direct my steps. When I arrived at the oncologist's office, I was filling out paperwork. As I was sitting there with my mom and sister, an old friend walked in with his wife. He is a strong

Christian man. As soon as he saw me, he hugged me and asked if I was there to see the doctor. I explained that I was. I knew from that point on that there would be more prayers for me.

I met with the oncologist, who reviewed my test results. He sat with my mom and me and explained that I would require surgery and that he would perform the surgery if I wanted him to.

I must be honest and say that I was probably in shock up until this point. I had to have so many tests. At this point I was nervous as I had lived 42 years without ever having any type of surgery, and I was facing the prospect of having major surgery. My surgery was scheduled for the next Friday, October 29, 2005.

The day arrived for my surgery, and I had a migraine. So much stress and not eating the night before the surgery had taken its toll. I arrived at the hospital with my husband, mom and dad, brother, sisters, and best friend. When it was time for me to go in to be prepped, my whole family stood up and formed a circle. We held hands while my brother prayed for my safekeeping and a successful surgery.

The surgery took longer than expected, and my family was told that I had cancer. My doctor took my mom and husband into a room to tell them the news. My mom told me they both broke down, but they decided together that my mom would tell the rest of the family because Jerry was unable to talk about it at that point. I was finally brought to my room. I was still groggy from the anesthesia, but as I was wheeled into my room, I could see in the dim light my family surrounding my bed. My husband Jerry leaned over and with tears in his eyes he whispered to me how much he loved me. He then told me that they had found cancer in one of my ovaries. As tears trickled out of my eyes, my dad leaned over and whispered in my ear that he would trade places with me if he could.

I did not realize that while my family was waiting for me to come out of recovery they had already made a list of who would be staying with me each night in the hospital, as they were going to take turns. When my sister Sherry stayed with me, she helped me bathe. My brother Cliff and my nephew Jon stayed with me another night. You never realize how much love your family has for you until they sacrifice their time and energy to help you get better. I felt so humbled by my family's love and caring attention.

Looking back now, I realized that everyone around me was in shock. I know there are certain steps that most people go through when they find out they have cancer. It starts with anger at God and asking "Why me?" It then moves to feeling sorry for yourself because it is you, then on to depression and many other emotions that are hard to deal with. I honestly never experienced any of those emotions. My first thought was what do I need to do to fully recover. So began my amazing journey.

I think that cancer is often harder on the loved ones around you. The one with cancer is often so involved in fighting the disease. Your loved ones often feel helpless in the fight. They struggle with how they can help you. They often don't realize that their just being there and praying for you daily is the best medicine they can give.

When my oncologist came to see me to explain the results, he told me I had stage IC ovarian cancer. I asked him what he recommended for my treatment. He said he thought I should have six chemo treatments to kill any cancer cells he may have missed during the surgery. I agreed; then began the long process of recovery from the surgery so that I would be ready for chemo.

Since my husband worked during the week, we decided that I would stay with my parents during the week so they could take care of me and that I would go home on the weekends to be with my husband. I must say my mom and dad were the best. I could not have done it without them. Mom made sure I ate well in order to gain back some of the weight I had lost during my surgery and recovery. We started walking at the high school track in the afternoons and sitting on their front porch in the evenings. On the weekends my husband Jerry would stop by and pick me up to take me home. He did all the grocery shopping and housecleaning and took care of our dog. My dog even mourned when I was not at home. I was truly blessed. God had much bigger plans for me.

I decided before my chemo treatments started that I would shave my head. One of my fears was that I would be standing in the shower and a large clump of my hair would fall out in my hands and I would be devastated. So I made an appointment with my hairdresser to have my head shaved. Another thing I did not realize when I was in surgery was that my family had discussed shaving their heads when it came time for me to have chemo treatments. They did not want me to be alone during that devastating process. I have heard it said that a woman's hair is her crowning glory. You don't realize how very true that is until you shave it off.

My appointment with the hairdresser arrived; my mom and sister Diane went with me. My sister brought her camera and a bottle of champagne. My mom decided she would shave her head first before I had to shave mine. She will never know how much that meant to me to have her show her support in that way. They made it an adventure filled with laughter and the sharing of memories that will live with me forever. My hairdresser gave my mom a mohawk before she shaved all her hair off, and we took pictures. When it came time to shave my head, my hairdresser cried because she had been giving me perms and cutting my hair for years, and she was getting ready to cut all my curls off. I think it was more devastating to her at the time than it was for me. She shaved one side of my head; then we laughed and took more pictures. As a final salute to the loss of hair, we raised our glasses in a toast.

When I arrived home, my husband and dog greeted us at the front door. I felt so naked without my hair. I kept touching my head in disbelief, as my head had never been that smooth. My husband walked up to me with tears in his eyes and told me how much he loved me and how beautiful I was.

We had another head-shaving party at my mom and dad's house. My brother Cliff brought his hair clippers and shaved designs on my sister Diane's head (and of course we took pictures). Then I got to shave my brother's head. Diane was always there to record each event with pictures. In the meantime my middle sister shaved my niece Rachel's hair off and she was a senior in high school. She attended her senior prom with very little hair. She had long beautiful brown hair that reached to the middle of her back. All her friends at school thought she was ill when she shaved her hair. In my eyes she was more beautiful then than she had ever been in her life.

My dad went to his hairdresser one day when I was staying with them. He didn't tell Mom or me what he intended to do. He told the hairdresser he wanted her to shave his head. She said, "Do you want a level 1 or level 2 shave?" That means the level of hair you want to shave off. My Dad told her to give him a "0." No hair. She asked him several times if he was sure before she shaved him bald.

My nephews, David, Jake, and Jon, were 15, 8, and 7 at the time I was diagnosed. I was afraid I would scare them with my not having hair, as they had always known me with long curly hair. They took it all in stride. My oldest nephew, David, let me play golf with him. When my hair starting growing back, my nephew, Jake, called me Aunt Diane because with my short hair I resembled my oldest sister. My nephew, Jon, made a bear for me. He drew it on paper, and my mom helped him sew it together. We called him "Irregular Bear" because his arms and legs were different sizes and his head was not totally round. Jon wanted a pocket sewn on front with a heart-shaped button. In the pocket, he printed a note that read, "I love you, Aunt Bren." To this day that bear means so much to me, as it shows the love that my nephew had for me.

I have many funny stories about this time. I believe if you can't see the humor in the situation, it will be tougher on you in the long run. One of the funniest stories was when we were at my mom and dad's house one morning and the UPS delivery guy showed up to deliver a package. We heard a knock on the door. Mom thought he was at the back door, and dad thought he was at the front. Dad stuck his bald head out the front door, and Mom met the guy at the back door with no hat or wig on her head. The UPS guy must have thought we were some type of cult, as he took off running to his truck when he saw my dad with his bald head sticking out the front door and my mom answering the door with her bald head.

After we all had our heads shaved, we picked a Saturday when all my family was in town and my husband was available. We spent 5 hours taking pictures of all of us bald. Those are my most treasured memories. The family I love dearly shaved their heads in support of me. Each time I look at those pictures I realize that it is not the hair that matters. It's the love that shines from the heart when you see the family you love so much without their hair. How can you measure that much love? I don't think that is possible.

After my leave of absence for surgery ended, I returned to full-time work except on the weeks that I had chemo treatments. I thought returning to work would be the most difficult time, and I approached that day with much trepidation. You see, my crowning glory was gone. I had shaved off all my hair and had purchased several wigs to wear. You always think that everyone will be able to tell that you have on a wig. Of course everyone at work already knew I would lose my hair, but I still had this idea in my head that they didn't know. And I feared I would have to face people who didn't know I had cancer, and people would point and whisper about the lady with no hair or the funny-looking wig. I had lost 8 pounds during my leave, so very few of my clothes fit. Everything just hung on my body.

When I walked in that first day back at work, my boss, Brad, had a new boss who he was meeting with that day. When I walked in, he came over and gave me a big bear hug. I say that because my boss is 6'4". He engulfed me in this huge hug, and tears filled my eyes. I knew at that point that I would be okay coming back to work. My boss was an attorney, so he is normally very stoic and reserved. You could tell he was thrilled that I was back, and that was exactly what I needed. I received more hugs that day than ever before. The support they showed me meant the world to me. I often laughed and joked about my various hats and wigs. One day around Christmas I received a Christmas hat from one of my good friends at work. It had white fur around the brim and a long red pipe cleaner sticking out of the center with a white fur ball on the end. When I walked, the white ball on the top wobbled back and forth. I went in and out of my boss's office. He acted as though I didn't have anything unusual on my head. Another day, I wore a flower pot hat that my aunt and cousins had sent to me during my recovery. The hat was in the shape of a flower pot with big, long-stemmed flowers sticking out of the top. My boss again just walked by my desk, told me good morning, and went right into his office as if I didn't have anything unusual on my head. From that point on I wore some rather unusual hats just to see if I could get a reaction from him.

One of the toughest things about chemo is that it can affect your memory. The reason this was tough for me was that my memory was one of the things that my boss always complimented me on. It was very difficult for me to remember things he asked me to do. Often when he asked me to do something, I forgot it as soon as I walked out of his office. I started carrying a notepad with me every time I went into his office. I wrote everything down. It helped me to remember things. I don't think he ever noticed the difference in my lapses in memory. By the way, my memory improved after my chemo treatments stopped. It took many months, but it did improve.

I had six chemotherapy treatments. My mom sat with me through them all. I also had a girlfriend who came and sat with me. She would show up with French toast or bacon and pancakes for us to eat during my treatments. Because of the chemicals injected into my body, it was hard for me to be hungry for anything. Everything I ate had a chemical, metallic taste. But Jan would always bring me something to eat. My mom always packed a bag with snacks for me. On those days, we sat and talked and shared many memories.

It had become a tradition for me to cook dressing for our Thanksgiving holiday. I am from Louisiana, so everything I cook has a Cajun flavor. This was the first year that I did not have the energy to cook. My mom, sister Sherry, and older sister Diane did the cooking. It was odd not helping with any of the cooking. We celebrated Thanksgiving with family and friends. Christmas was really special. We draw names for gifts in our family. My brother had drawn my sister's name. Her gift was framed pictures of our family photo session, "Bald is Beautiful." When you see the love that shines through when your family has no hair, it is an amazing thing. It puts everything else in perspective. Everything else is small stuff compared to your journey with cancer.

The week of my third treatment, my grandmother passed away. This was a sad time, as I had not been able to visit with her in the nursing home since my surgery and chemo treatments. I had a treatment on Friday. On Saturday, I rode with my parents for 6 hours back to Lake Charles, Louisiana, to attend the funeral. Hurricane Rita had just hit the Gulf Coast and Lake Charles in particular. There was so much damage in the area where my grandmother would be buried that there were no hotels within a hundred miles. We had to stay in a hotel in Lafayette, an hour and a half away. To complete the funeral arrangements we had to drive back and forth, to and from our hotel for several days. My grandmother's request was that her granddaughters, nieces, and great niece be pallbearers at her funeral. That Tuesday I was able to be a pallbearer for my grandmother. I can still picture my sisters, cousins, and niece all dressed in black carrying my grandmother's casket. It had been an emotional journey.

The fourth treatment came along. I was more tired than usual. I did not realize that I had a bleeding ulcer. On the Tuesday after treatment, I woke up not feeling well. I could not walk without getting dizzy. I called my doctor, and the nurse asked me to come in immediately. My blood count was so low they checked me directly into the hospital from the physician's office. I was given two pints of blood and scheduled for a scope. They found the ulcer, cauterized it, and then released me on Friday. I was back at work the following Monday.

I never missed a treatment until the last one. My blood counts were too low. I had worn my special flower pot hat for the final one. I had to go home and try again in a week. I arrived for my treatment again, and still my counts were too low. Each time I had to call my husband to tell him it was postponed again. I could tell he was more worried than ever before. Finally, I arrived the next week, and my counts were good enough to do the treatment. I called my husband to let him know. He just broke down and cried.

That evening after my treatment I went home and sat down with my husband. I had not realized until that moment how hard the treatments and cancer had been on him. He had been trying to be strong for me, but at the same time he sat on the couch every night worrying and praying. I finally understood what this whole process had done to him. In his being strong for me he had been holding in all his worries and fears. That night he broke down and cried over his fear of losing me. I explained to him that if God saw fit to take me from this world, I was ready, and that is what gave me peace through the whole process. Being human, my husband told me that I might be ready for that time, but he certainly wasn't ready for me to go. I explained to him that he needed to talk to me about his fears and worries because I could not make it through this journey without him.

I completed my chemo treatments in March 2006. I had my 1-year check-up in March 2007, and I continue to improve every day. This cancer journey has taken me to places I never dreamed. I consider it a blessing from God that I have taken this walk with Him. I thank my family, friends, and all those who prayed for me during this time and have continued to celebrate the many milestones that have occurred since then. There were many who prayed for me whom I have never met. I hope one day to meet each of you and thank you personally for the prayers. I could not have made this journey without you.

I believe God allowed this to happen to me for a reason, and prayer played a large part in my healing. It made me and the people around me more aware of the wonderful thing He gives us called *life*. This life I live on earth is by no means the best place I will ever see. One day God will call me "home," and what a blessed place that will be. What a blessed life I have lived.

Brenda Edwards

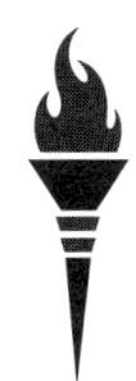

Resources

Books

Becton, Randy. *Everyday Strength: A Cancer Patient's Guide to Spiritual Survival.* Baker Books, 2006.

Clegg, Holly; Miletello, Gerald, MD. *Eating Well Through Cancer: Easy Recipes and Recommendations During and After Treatments.* The Cookbook Marketplace, 2006.

Connor, Kristine; Langford, Lauren. *Ovarian Cancer: Your Guide to Taking Control.* Patient Center Guides, 2003.

Davis, Martha; Eshelman, Elizabeth Robbins; McKay, Matthew. *The Relaxation/Stress Reduction Workbook.* New Harbinger Press, 2000.

Dyer, Diana. *A Dietitian's Cancer Story.* Swan Press, 2002.

Groopman, Jerome, MD. *The Anatomy of Hope: How People Prevail in the Face of Illness.* Random House, 2005.

Harpham, Wendy Schlessel, MD. *Becky and the Worry Cup: A Children's Book About a Parent's Cancer.* Perennial, 1997.

Harpham, Wendy Schlessel, MD. *Diagnosis: Cancer: Your Guide to the First Months of Healthy Survivorship.* W.W. Norton, 2003.

Harpham, Wendy Schlessel, MD. *Happiness in a Storm: Facing Illness and Embracing Life as a Healthy Survivor.* W.W. Norton, 2005

Harpham, Wendy Schlessel, MD. *When a Parent Has Cancer: A Guide to Caring for Your Children.* Harper, 2004.

Harvey, John R., PhD. *Total Relaxation: Healing Practices for Body, Mind & Spirit* (with CD). Kodansha America, 1998.

Holland, Jimmie C., MD; Lewis, Sheldon Holland. *The Human Side of Cancer: Living with Hope, Coping with Uncertainty.* HarperCollins, 2000.

Montz, F.J.; Bristow, Robert E.; Anastasia, Paula J. *A Guide to Survivorship for Women with Ovarian Cancer.* The Johns Hopkins University Press, 2005.

Pacini, Greg. *Journey Beyond Diagnosis: Support During and After Illness for Survivors and Those Who Love and Care for Them.* Reedy Press, 2005.

Schwartz, Anna L., PhD; Armstrong, Lance (Foreword). *Cancer Fitness: Exercise Programs for Patients and Survivors.* Fireside, 2004.

Silver, Alex, Emily, and Anna Rose. *Our Mom Is Getting Better.* American Cancer Society, 2007.

Silver, Alex, Emily, and Anna Rose. *Our Dad Is Getter Better.* American Cancer Society, 2007.

Silver, Julie K., MD. *After Cancer Treatment: Heal Faster, Better, Stronger.* The Johns Hopkins University Press, 2006.

Weldon, Glen. *Dietary Options for Cancer Survivors.* American Institute for Cancer Research, 2002. (This book can be ordered through the American Institute for Cancer Research's Web site: www.aicr.org. This Web site is also an excellent resource for up-to-date information on nutrition and cancer and a good source for recipes.)

Web Sites for Information and Support

National Ovarian Cancer Coalition, www.ovarian.org, 888-682-7426

Conversations (Newsletter for Ovarian Cancer Patients), www.ovarian-news.org, 806-355-2565

American Association of Sex Educators, Counselors and Therapists, www.aasect.org, 319-895-8407

American Cancer Society, www.cancer.org, 800-ACS-2345

American Psychosocial Oncology Society, www.apos-society.org

American Society of Clinical Oncology, www.asco.org

People Living with Cancer, www.plwc.org, 888-651-3038

Cancer Care, Inc., www.cancercare.org, 212-712-8080

Cancer Net, www.cancernet.gov

Cancer Trials, www.cancer.gov/clinical_trials

Council of State Administrators of Vocational Rehabilitation, www.rehabnetwork.org, 301-654-8414

Gilda's Club, www.glidasclub.org, 888-GILDA-4-U

Lance Armstrong Foundation, www.laf.org, 512-236-8820

Look Good…Feel Better, www.lookgoodfeelbetter.org, 800-395-LOOK

National Cancer Institute, www.cancer.gov, 800-4-CANCER

National Center for Complementary and Alternative Medicine,
    www.nccam.nih.gov, 888-644-6226

National Coalition for Cancer Survivorship, www.canceradvocacy.org,
    877-NCCS-YES

National Family Caregivers Association, www.nfcacares.org, 800-896-3650

Oncology Nursing Society, www.ons.org, 866-257-4557

SHARE (Self-Help for Women with Breast or Ovarian Cancer),
    www.sharecancersupport.org, 212-719-1204

The Well Spouse Foundation, www.wellspouse,org, 800-838-0879

The Wellness Community, www.wellness-community.org, 888-793-WELL

Women's Center for Mind-Body Health, www.womensmindbodyhealth.info,
    650-559-9597

Young Survival Coalition, www.youngsurvival.org, 212-206-6610

Other Resources

Shibashi

Description: A gentle, flowing active-range-of-motion exercise, combined
    with positive intentions, similar to tai chi, but simpler. The routine is
    about 12 minutes in duration, and can be performed semi-seated in a
    hospital bed, seated, or standing.

Resource: DVD demonstrating Shibashi in standing and in adapted versions,
    produced by the Healing Environment Program at Baylor University
    Medical Center. To order, call the Charles A. Sammons Cancer Center at
    Dallas: 214-820-3136.

Aromablends

    Dr. Judy Griffith, www.aromahealthtexas.com

Relaxation CDs and Audiotapes

    Nischala Joy Devi, www.abundantwellbeing.com

    Dr. Herbert Bensen, Mind/Body Institute, www.mbmi.org

    Relaxation Music, www.mozarteffect.com